Michael van Straten

detox super

whitecap

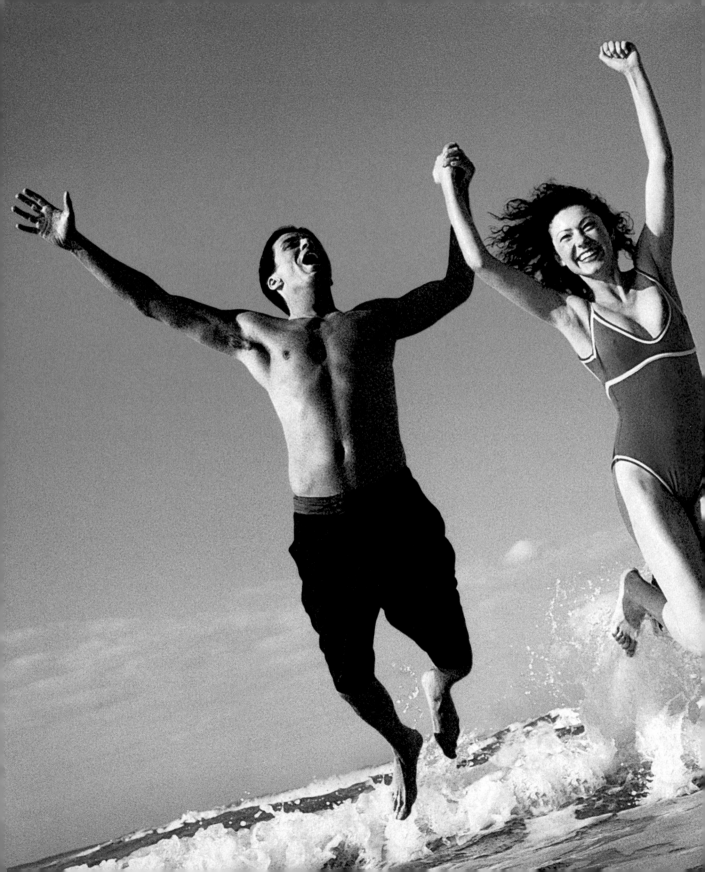

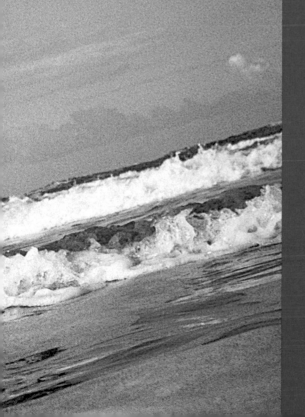

contents

introduction

There's nothing new about detoxing—it's as old as man himself—and has been part of our healing heritage for many thousands of years. The whole practice of detoxing has grown out of the ancient concepts of fasting—and fasting is the key to both physical and spiritual cleansing.

Almost every religion in the world uses fasting in some form to increase spiritual awareness and sharpen the powers of mental agility. Sadly, in our modern world detoxing has become a quick fix—an instant solution to the problems of pain and over-indulgence. After 364 days of junk food, too much alcohol, and no exercise, you can't expect much benefit from one day of fasting on nothing but water and herb tea.

This book will introduce you to the true principles of fasting and detoxing—which means preparing for your detox, following your chosen regimen, whether it's a 24- or 48-hour or three-day program, and, after that, using an eight-day menu planner which returns you gradually to "normal" eating.

For those of you whose "normal" eating is a bit of a disaster, you'll also find a 14-day guide to a balanced, healthy, but enjoyable eating plan which you can follow for the rest of your life.

Everyone needs the occasional treat—a traditional Christmas feast and the over-indulgence of Thanksgiving—but these don't matter that much since it's what you do most of the time that's really important.

Different problems require different solutions, and for this reason, the book is divided into several sections: Super Health Detox, Super Energy Detox and Super Radiance Detox, each of which focusses on a specific area of concern.

Detoxing for health is the foundation on which to build a better immune system, and your body's defence against many life-threatening and life-disrupting illnesses.

Detoxing for energy may not seem that important in the scheme of things, but millions of you wake up every morning exhausted and worn out. In fact, fatigue is one of the most common reasons for consulting a physician. Poor eating habits and the enormous stress involved in trying to fit work, family, and friends into the hectic 24/7 world of the 21st century are a great drain on your body's energy resources, which results in chronic fatigue and serious damage to your immune system. Reducing the toxic load and improving the standard of your daily nutrition will make a highly significant difference in a very short time.

Detoxing for radiance is about much more than getting rid of the odd blemish on your face. To look radiant on the outside you must be radiant on the inside, too. It's this combination that achieves super radiance. Lustrous skin, hair, and nails are the obvious benefits, but this type of inner beauty is the result of good digestion, an efficient heart and circulatory system, strong bones, and pain-free joints. All these can be achieved by eating more of the best food and less of the worst. Excessive alcohol, caffeine, and nicotine aren't good for the skin—or anything else, for that matter. So quit smoking and be sensible about the others.

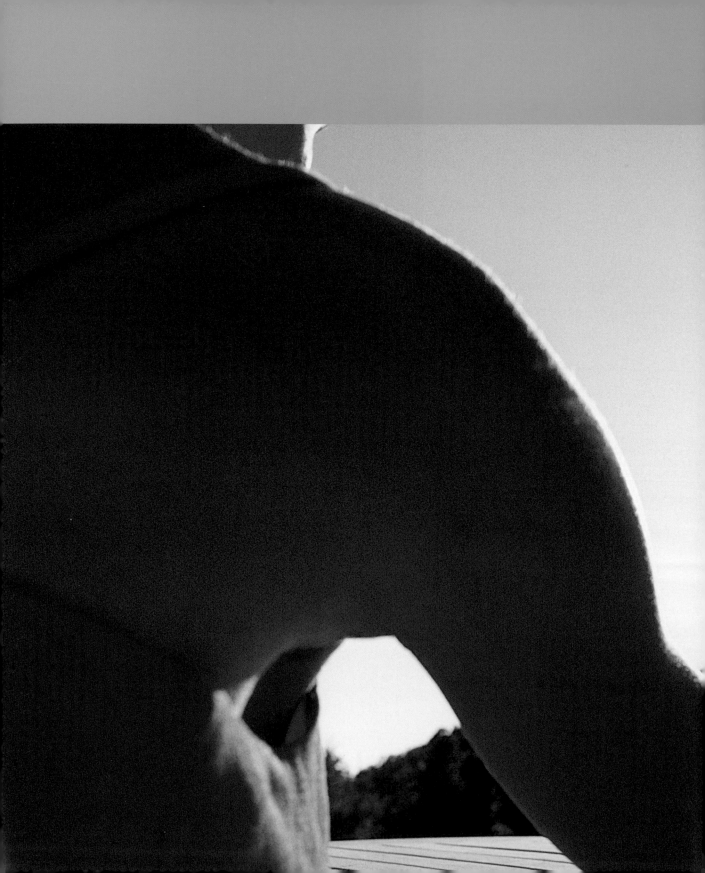

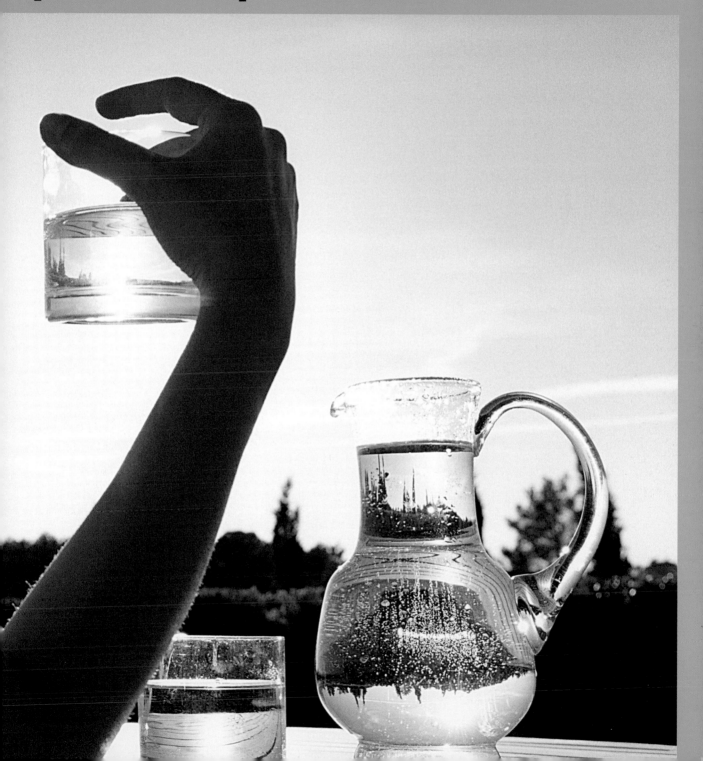

the search for super health

Many factors affect your health but there are only two over which you have no control whatsoever. You can't choose your parents, so you're stuck with whatever genetic influences they pass on. Nor can you plan for acts of God. That said, the vast majority of other health problems you're likely to have are, to a greater or lesser extent, in your own hands.

After 40 years in practice as a naturopath, osteopath, and acupuncturist, there is almost nothing that people do regarding their health that surprises me any more. But I am still constantly amazed at the way in which people adopt the most extreme attitudes and practices when it comes to health-related issues.

On the one hand, there is a sizeable proportion of people who never give a second thought to what they eat or drink, how they live their lives, or what detrimental impact their lifestyles can have on both their minds and their bodies. They totally ignore even the most sensible of health warnings. They simply don't care or can't be bothered.

At the opposite end of the scale are those who adopt, hook, line, and sinker, every extreme health idea that's ever promoted. These are the health fanatics, the small minority who follow the most draconian of regimes in pursuit of the holy grail of thinness and eternal youth. It's this group of extremists that worries me most, as they are far more likely to suffer long-term health damage than those with a relaxed attitude to diet and lifestyle. These health fanatics, mostly young women, are easy prey for every new, high-profile health guru who turns up in the media. They end up on diets that fail to supply the most basic nutritional needs, they frequently over-exercise, and they are nearly always too thin. In addition, they subject themselves to ridiculous therapies, bogus allergy tests, and questionable, if not frankly dangerous, practices like colonic irrigation. As a result, they run the risk of developing a host of health problems ranging from eating disorders to osteoporosis.

What makes this scenario even more worrying is when these extremists apply their latest health craze to their children and decide to bring them up on unrealistic, very restricted, and highly dangerous diets.

This is not the way to super health but an almost certain way to a life of ill health and unhappiness. The pressure that these extreme regimes put upon friends, families, and partners is a major factor, too. Normal social life becomes impossible, the pleasure of an enjoyable meal at a convivial table is lost forever, and an insupportable strain is placed on any normal relationship.

There are great dangers to the health of our society in the way many people live, but you can minimize these risks for yourself with a little bit of self-discipline, some very modest lifestyle changes, and the inclusion of a wider selection of the most delicious foods. So dump any forms of extremism. That's not the way to super health. Instead, just follow my simple Super Health Detox plan and give your body the tools it needs to maintain a long, happy, and disease-free life.

time to detox?

Everyone, no matter how super-healthy they may be, would benefit from the occasional detox. But some people's need is more serious. To find out how much you need Super Health Detox, answer these questions – truthfully, as the only person you'll be cheating is yourself – then work out your score.

1 How many times a week do you eat breakfast?
- **A** Every day.
- **B** Most days if I've got time.
- **C** Breakfast? Do coffee and cookies at 11 o'clock count?

2 You know you should be eating five portions of fruit and vegetables a day. What does that consist of?
- **A** Apples, oranges, bananas, greens, salads – any I can lay my hands on.
- **B** Will five grapes and some french fries do?
- **C** Who says I have to eat five pieces of fruit a day? I hate the stuff.

3 How much of the food you eat consists of processed food like burgers, sausages, and frozen TV dinners?
- **A** None – I like cooking proper meals.
- **B** Not much – but I do eat them three or four times a week when I'm busy.
- **C** Most of it – I don't have time to cook.

4 When you use oil or fat for cooking, what type is it?
- **A** Good olive oil.
- **B** Sunflower or other seed oil.
- **C** Butter, lard, or hard margarine.

5 How often do you eat oily fish like sardines, salmon, and mackerel?
- **A** At least once a week – I know it's good for me.
- **B** Probably not that often, but I know I should eat more.
- **C** I don't think they sell them at our burger place.

6 What type of milk do you normally buy?
- **A** Mostly skim – I'm watching my weight.
- **B** 2 percent – it doesn't taste as good as ordinary milk but I know it's healthier.
- **C** Full fat – the others are all revolting.

7 Bread is the staff of life. Which do you normally choose?
- **A** Whole-wheat – the fiber keeps me regular.
- **B** A variety, I like all sorts.
- **C** I never touch bread, it's fattening.

8 Do you (check as many as you like)
Smoke?
Drink more than 14 drinks (women) or 21 drinks (men) of alcohol a week?
Take sleeping pills/tranquilizers/anti-depressants?
Use recreational drugs?

9 Which of the following sums up your exercise pattern?
- **A** I exercise loads – I practically live at the gym.
- **B** I don't do as much as I should, but I do play tennis/football or kick a ball around with the kids three or four times a week.
- **C** Well, I walk from the car to the supermarket/bar.

10 How often do you make time to do something you want?

A At least once a week – I know I need to spoil myself occasionally.

B Not that often, but I probably get a break once a month or so.

C Never – my job/the kids/the home are far too demanding.

11 Have you ever suffered from constipation?

A No.

B From time to time, but it has never been a serious problem.

C I've had it for as long as I can remember.

12 The elevator's broken and you walk up three floors. How breathless are you?

A Not at all.

B A little, but it only lasts a couple of minutes.

C I think I'm dying and it takes 10 minutes to get my breath back.

13 How many times a year do you catch a cold or flu?

A Hardly ever.

B Two or three.

C I've lost count – if there's a bug around I get it.

14 How often do you get headaches (apart from migraine) and have to take painkillers?

A Once in a blue moon.

B Occasionally.

C Most days.

15 In the last twelve months, how often have you been prescribed antibiotics by your doctor?

A 2 or less.

B 3–5.

C I've lost count.

Score:

A – 1 point
B – 3 points
C or check – 5 points

Over 85 – start detoxing now and check your life insurance policy. This is not the time to buy War and Peace – you may not be around long enough to finish reading it!

60–85 – all is not lost. A few changes to your eating and lifestyle, a bit more exercise and you'll soon be in better health. Pay special attention to the rebuilding for health regime (see pages 32–35).

35–60 – you're doing a great job. You're probably eating well, taking some exercise, have a good understanding about how your body works, but are still having fun.

under 35 – you win the booby prize! You may be super healthy but your life is very dull. You're probably a food freak and a hypochondriac, worrying about everything you put in your mouth and the health risks of everything that's pleasurable in life. Lighten up and remember that in the concert of life there is no rehearsal. You might be a health fanatic but you could be struck by lightning tomorrow.

I'm sure you've worked it out by now, but all the As are the healthiest or correct answers, Bs not quite right, Cs and checks mean bad news.

cleansing for

Cleanliness is next to godliness so most people wash, bathe, or shower every day, but how often do you think about cleansing the inside? Apart from the toxic chemicals you absorb from the environment and from your food and drink, the body also produces its own waste. Much of this is eliminated naturally, but some remains in the body as unwanted chemical by-products and free radicals and these will all eventually harm your health. Fasting is a way of getting rid of them. It will also increase your blood's white-cell count, which will help boost your natural immunity and protect you from disease.

when should I detox?

As a naturopath I strongly advise the regular – ideally once a week – use of a twenty-four hour juice and water fast as a way of maintaining good health. If regular twenty-four hour fasting doesn't appeal to you, then a forty-eight hour regime, not more than once a month, is an extremely effective health-inducing body cleanser. I offer a structured forty-eight hour program, but if you want you could go for two days on just water and juices. If you do this, though, by the end of the second day you'll feel a certain amount of light-headedness, so it's advisable not to undertake strenuous physical activity, drive, or use dangerous machinery.

For a seasonal clear-out, a three-day regime is ideal. It's also a great way to help your body recover from illness, but seek medical advice before starting if you've recently been ill. The three-day program consists largely of a combination of water, juices, clear soups, and some fresh fruit and vegetables. This fast is not suitable while you're working and should be scheduled when you can have at least one day to recover. For example, you could start at work on Friday, complete the fast on Saturday and Sunday, then have Monday as a day off.

health

side effects

The most common side effect of fasting is headache. This is caused partly by the drop in blood-sugar levels and the beginnings of elimination, but often it's caused by the body being deprived of caffeine. The more coffee you usually drink, the worse the headache is likely to be. Don't resort to painkillers; simply drink lots more water and it will pass.

During forty-eight hour or three-day fasts you may also get what naturopaths call a "healing crisis" – a coated tongue, bad breath, increased temperature, sweating, tremors, and general aches and pains. This is traditionally believed to be caused by the sudden release of accumulated toxins from the body. We now know that it's the result of the natural bacteria in the gut dying off and releasing chemicals which are then absorbed by the gut wall. Don't worry if any of these things happen to you; they're a good sign.

take care

If you've recently been ill you should check with your doctor before starting any fast. Similarly, if you have an underlying illness like diabetes or you are on prescribed medication that needs to be taken with food – non-steroidal anti-inflammatories, for example – you especially need to exercise caution and consult your regular physician. Take care if you suffer from migraine, as fasting can trigger attacks, and although short detox periods are fine during pregnancy and breastfeeding, you should not do more than three days.

And to do the best you can for your body, during your detox try to consume only organic produce and, if possible, make your own juices. Now's the time to invest in that juicer!

the extras

Detoxing is not simply giving up food. You need to take care about what and how much you drink and about how much exercise you need. In addition, my experience has shown that taking some commonly available food supplements while you detox will ensure your body benefits to the maximum.

what to drink

First thing in the morning make up a pitcher of Parsley Tea (see recipe, page 189), keep it in the fridge and drink small glasses regularly throughout the day. This gentle diuretic will help to speed up the detoxifying and cleansing processes, so make sure you drink it all.

You can drink as much water and herb or weak green tea as you like, but don't add milk or any form of sweetener. And you must not consume fizzy water, canned drinks, alcohol, black tea, coffee, or any sweetened drinks. This includes sugar-free commercial products, which contain artificial sweeteners.

the supplements

No matter whether you choose to do a twenty-four hour cleansing detox, or the forty-eight hour or three-day versions, you can improve the efficiency of the program and support your body's whole system by taking the appropriate supplements every day.

for general well-being

During all these programs you will be consuming far less food than normal and even though the recommended foods will provide an abundance of nutrients, it is important to give your body an extra supportive boost of vitamins and minerals to avoid any possible deficiencies and to guarantee optimum levels. For this reason you should take:

▶ A high-potency multi-vitamin and mineral supplement (choose one of the reputable brand leaders);
▶ 500mg vitamin C, three times a day. If you can find it, use ester-C, which many leading manufacturers now include in their products as it is non-acidic and less likely to cause digestive upsets – especially important while you're eating less food.

▶ A one-a-day standardized extract of cynarin – from globe artichokes. This stimulates liver function and helps the body eliminate fat-soluble substances stored in the liver.

for bowel function

Maintaining proper and regular bowel function is especially important during a detox as you will have a much lower fiber intake than normal.

▶ To stimulate, improve, and maintain bowel function take 1–2 tablespoons of oatbran or ground psyllium seed every night while you follow the plans and, for best results, start the day before. Both provide water-soluble fiber – better described as smoothage rather than roughage.

for a weak immune system

If your immune system has obviously been under par, then detoxing will help boost your natural immunity. But if you've been ill, take these additional supplements:

▶ Vitamin C and zinc – vital for a healthy immune system. They're best taken together in a lozenge;
▶ Echinacea – one of the most effective herbs for short-term immunity boosting;
▶ Probiotics – beneficial bacteria that are a key factor in strengthening your body's defense mechanisms.

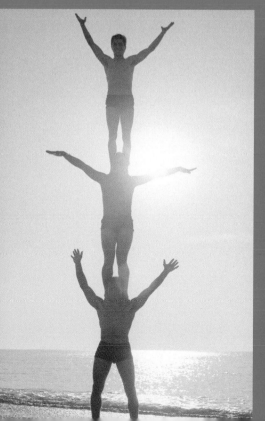

rest and exercise

Rest while you're detoxing but don't turn into a couch potato. Staying in bed a little longer in the morning, having a catnap during the day, and going to bed a bit earlier in the evening are all sensible.

However, you also need some physical activity to stimulate your metabolism, hormones, blood flow, and digestive function. Take two or three short walks – not more than 10–15 minutes each day – whatever the weather and dress appropriately. Don't jog, run, go to the gym, or clean the house. Over-exertion will drain your energy, produce a lot of toxic chemical by-products, and inhibit your cleansing regime.

twenty-four hour cleansing

If you've had a week of over-indulgence in food or alcohol, this twenty-four hour Cleansing for Health fast will flush out your system and revitalize your mind and body. Even if you're not suffering from any self-inflicted damage, it's an excellent way of compensating for the unavoidable environmental hazards we're constantly exposed to and will give you a short, sharp, good-health boost.

This twenty-four hour detox can easily be incorporated into even the most hectic of lifestyles. Though best done on a non-working day, most people in reasonably good health can manage the fast even while working. Used on a regular, weekly, basis, it represents a huge investment in your good health.

on waking	A large glass of hot water with a thick slice of organic unwaxed lemon
breakfast	A large glass of hot water with a thick slice of organic unwaxed lemon A mug of Ginger Tea (see recipe, page 189)
mid-morning	A large glass of hot water with a thick slice of organic unwaxed lemon
lunch	A large glass of Tomato Juice, Celery, and Celery Leaf Blend (see recipe, page 188) A mug of Ginger Tea (see recipe, page 189)
mid-afternoon	A large glass of hot water with a thick slice of organic unwaxed lemon
supper	Kiwi and Pineapple Juice (see recipe, page 188) A mug of Ginger Tea (see recipe, page 189)
evening	Orange Juice and Almond Blend (see recipe, page 188)
bedtime	A mug of camomile tea (any reputable brand) with a teaspoon of organic honey

forty-eight hour cleansing

If a one-day-a-week detox doesn't appeal to you, you might prefer a forty-eight hour regime that you do once a month. Start by following the twenty-four hour Cleansing for Health fast, then for the next twenty-four hours have:

on waking   A large glass of hot water with a thick slice of organic unwaxed lemon

breakfast   A large glass of hot water with a thick slice of organic unwaxed lemon
An orange
Half a pink grapefruit
A slice of cantaloupe
A mug of camomile tea

mid-morning   A large glass of hot water with a thick slice of organic unwaxed lemon

lunch   A large plate of mixed raw red and yellow bell pepper, cucumber, carrot, radishes, tomatoes, celery, and broccoli, with a handful of chopped fresh parsley and a drizzle of extra-virgin olive oil and lemon juice
A large glass of unsweetened apple juice
A mug of mint tea

mid-afternoon   A large glass of hot water with a thick slice of organic unwaxed lemon

supper   A large bowl of fresh fruit salad, to include apple, pear, grapes, mango, and some berries – but no banana
A handful of raisins – make sure to chew them very slowly – and a handful of fresh, unsalted cashew nuts
A glass of unsalted mixed vegetable juice (any reputable brand)

evening   A large glass of hot water with a thick slice of organic unwaxed lemon

bedtime   A mug of camomile tea with a teaspoon of organic honey

three-day cleansing

A three-day detox is quite a serious undertaking. Though not strictly speaking a fast, other than on the first day, you will feel noticeable side effects so this program is definitely best done when you are not working. Because of your very low calorie intake, you will certainly feel quite light-headed by the end of day 2 and even more so during day 3. Any severe headaches will pass and towards the end you may begin to feel euphoric.

Because this is a cleansing regime, as your body steps up its eliminating processes it's likely that you will develop unpleasant breath, a coated tongue, and will urinate more frequently than normal. It's essential that you keep your liquid intake at the recommended level to replace any fluid you have lost and to stimulate further elimination. It's unlikely that you will have any unusual problems with gas, but even though you're eating much less bulk than normal you may find that your bowels are more active, especially in the latter part of day 3.

Take care when you return to normal eating after this three-day plan. I recommend you follow the eight-day return to normal eating program (see pages 20–23), but if you don't have time for that just make sure you don't overload your digestive system. Eat little and often, avoid all animal protein, high-fat and fried foods, and apart from yogurt, avoid all other dairy products. On day 4 you will need to drink at least one and a half quarts of fluid. You can eat any fruit and vegetables and introduce some starchy food in the form of oats, whole-wheat bread, rice, and pasta. A small amount of grilled, poached, or steamed white fish would be fine, but don't have shellfish, seafood, or oily fish.

Days 1 and 2, follow the Forty-Eight Hour Cleansing program. Day 3:

on waking A large glass of hot water with a thick slice of organic unwaxed lemon

breakfast A large glass of hot water with a thick slice of organic unwaxed lemon
A carton of organic low-fat live yogurt with a teaspoon of honey, 2 teaspoons of raisins and 2 teaspoons of chopped hazelnuts
A glass of half-orange, half-grapefruit juice

mid-morning A large glass of Carrot, Apple, and Celery juice (see recipe, page 187)
4 dried apricots
4 prunes

lunch A large glass of hot water with a thick slice of organic unwaxed lemon
Carrot and Red Cabbage Salad (see recipe, page 239)
A mug of mint tea

mid-afternoon A glass of any unsweetened fruit juice

supper A mixture of chopped steamed leek, cabbage, spinach, and kale, drizzled with olive oil, lemon juice, and a generous sprinkling of ground nutmeg
A glass of unsweetened red grape juice
A mug of lime-blossom (linden or tilia) tea

evening 4 prunes
4 dates
A small bunch of blue or purple grapes

bedtime A cup of green tea with two rice crackers

eight-day return to normal eating

If you've managed to do the full three-day detox, you're obviously serious about getting your health back on target. Now follow this eight-day plan to reaccustom your body to normal eating and maximize the health benefits. The plan provides large quantities of protective and health-promoting anti-oxidants, which are good for your heart, circulation, blood pressure, and cholesterol. They also give your body a valuable cancer-protective boost, while at the same time providing an abundance of the essential basic nutrients.

If you've only done the twenty-four hour program, then this plan is pretty much optional, but I do suggest you try to follow it for just two days. If you've done the forty-eight hour program, then you should follow at least the first two days of the plan.

It's extremely important that you follow day 1 exactly as it's laid out, but the remaining seven days are more flexible and within each day you may switch light meals and main meals to suit your lifestyle. You can also switch whole days around, but don't mix meals from one day with meals from another as this upsets the balance of the eating plan.

keeping up your fluid intake

While you're doing this, you must keep your fluid intake at a minimum of one and a half quarts a day, but the same rules about canned drinks and commercial juices apply as for the detox programs. Many people find that once they've gotten into the habit of starting their day with hot water and lemon, it becomes a valuable addition to their normal regime. It avoids the early morning caffeine shot, stimulates the digestive system, and helps to get your bowels moving regularly.

And now that you've managed to reduce your caffeine intake, try to keep it down. There's nothing wrong with two or three cups a day of your favorite tea or good coffee, but more than this is not a long-term health benefit as excessive amounts of caffeine can be a factor in raising your blood pressure.

day 1

on waking   A large glass of hot water with a thick slice of organic unwaxed lemon

breakfast   A helping of fresh fruit salad consisting of apple, pear, grapes, mango, and pineapple with a carton of low-fat live yogurt and a tablespoon of good quality unsweetened muesli
A mug of any herb tea

mid-morning   6 dried apricots
A glass of unsweetened pineapple juice

lunch   A large bowl of Lettuce Soup (see recipe, page 229) with a chunk of My Easy Bread (see recipe, page 176) – no butter
A cup of any herb or green tea

mid-afternoon   An apple
A pear

supper   Pasta with Lettuce Pesto (see recipe, page 193)
A cup of any herb or green tea

day 2

on waking   A large glass of hot water with a thick slice of organic unwaxed lemon

breakfast   Half a pink grapefruit
Poached Egg and Tomato (see recipe, page 177)

light meal   An avocado and 2 tablespoons of cottage cheese
A large bunch of grapes

main meal   Cucumber and Strawberry Salad (see recipe, page 237)
Mixed Vegetable Stir-Fry with Rice (see recipe, page 192)

day 3

breakfast   A large peach with any seasonal berries

light meal   A large green salad of watercress, celery, raw spinach, basil, coriander, chicory, and dark lettuce like romaine, with a portion of steamed carrots, zucchini, peas, fava beans and corn, tossed in a scant teaspoon of butter, sprinkled with chopped mint

main meal   A bowl of Vegetable Soup (see recipe, page 229)
A large Stuffed Red Bell Pepper (see recipe, page 226)
2 pieces of fresh fruit – not bananas

day 4

breakfast   A large bowl of cherries or other seasonal berries with a carton of plain, low-fat live yogurt

light meal   A mixed green salad
Pasta all'Aglio e Olio (see recipe, page 197)

main meal   Tsatsiki (see recipe, page 238)
Grilled Chicken Breast on Iceberg Lettuce (see recipe, page 193) with grilled tomato and baby new potatoes boiled in their skins
A large peach

day 5

breakfast   Porridge Muesli (see recipe, page 176)
A banana

light meal   A whole-wheat pita bread filled with sliced hard-boiled egg, chopped tomato, cucumber, raw fennel, and shredded lettuce

main meal   Celery Salad (see recipe, page 238)
Baked Stuffed Trout (see recipe, page 195) served with warm snap beans tossed in a drizzle of olive oil and a squeeze of lemon juice and sprinkled with chopped green onions and parsley

day 6

breakfast   A large bunch of grapes

light meal   A bowl of Vegetable Soup (see recipe, page 229) with a whole-wheat roll
A selection of washed, sliced raw vegetables to include radishes, carrot, fennel, celery, and olives
A ripe pear

main meal   Veggie Curry with Rice (see recipe, page 195)
Tomato, Red Onion, and Beet Salad (see recipe, page 239)
2 kiwi fruit

day 7

breakfast   A selection of mixed soft fruits such as strawberries, raspberries, currants, apricots, and peaches

light meal   Tuna and Cottage-Cheese Stuffed Tomatoes (see recipe, page 196) with a small green salad and 2 slices of My Easy Bread (see recipe, page 176)

main meal   Stir-Fried Tofu with Vegetables and Noodles (see recipe, page 196)
A glass of Berry Smoothie (see recipe, page 189)

day 8

breakfast   2 organic free-range boiled eggs with 1 slice of whole-wheat toast and butter
A large glass of freshly squeezed orange juice

light meal   Mushrooms with Radicchio and Chicory (see recipe, page 193) with 1 slice of whole-wheat bread
An apple and a pear

main meal   Grapefruit, Peach and Mascarpone Salad (see recipe, page 239)
Grilled Salmon Steak (see recipe, page 197) served with boiled potatoes and any green vegetable you like
A matchbox-size piece of your favorite cheese with a stalk of celery, a handful of radishes, and 2 rye crispbreads

replenishing

You're doing well and your health is improving. You've detoxed and cleansed and now it's time to look to the longer term. Even if you haven't spent the last five years living on junk food and burning the candle at both ends, you probably haven't followed the most healthy of eating patterns. You've looked at some health and diet books and thought that living on a vegan or macrobiotic diet, going to your friends' for dinner with a brown paper bag full of mung beans, grated carrot, and a bottle of your own freshly made wheatgrass juice is not quite your cup of tea. So what else can you do?

the french paradox

You're now going to start replenishing your body's depleted stores of many of the essential nutrients. But you can put away the hair shirt and take a leaf out of nearly any French or Mediterranean cookbook.

In the early 1990s a French researcher spotted the surprising fact that although his countrymen (and women and children) ate mountains of runny cheese, munched their way through kilos of paté and foie gras, drank liters of wine and smoked hundreds of their unique cigarettes, they suffered 30 percent less heart disease than people living in northern Europe and the USA. And people in the south of France suffered 30 per cent less than the rest of their compatriots.

Though this phenomenon is now known as the French Paradox, the same sorts of results are apparent throughout the Mediterranean countries. What is more, recent studies have shown that men who had already suffered a heart attack and then switched to a Mediterranean diet cut their chances of a second attack by 70 percent. Not surprisingly this news has made the French Paradox even more exciting.

for health

Naturopaths like me have been advocating French and Mediterranean styles of eating for years. Prevention of heart disease is just one benefit. Less bowel cancer, fewer circulatory problems, fewer gallstones, and less osteoporosis and rheumatic disease are some others. That's because a Mediterranean diet

▶ is lower in saturated fatty acids – the animal fats that are a major contributor to heart disease

▶ is rich in polyunsaturated fatty acids from vegetable oils, which do not cause heart disease

▶ is very rich in mono-unsaturated fatty acids from olive oil, nuts, and seeds, which help the body to get rid of cholesterol and protect your heart and arteries

▶ is rich in dietary fiber, which improves digestion and bowel function and protects against some forms of cancer

▶ contains lots of chemicals called polyphenols from red wine, fruits, and vegetables, which are protective and anti-aging anti-oxidants

▶ consists of less red meat and far more fish and shellfish, which means less bad fat, more good fat and minerals – especially iodine, zinc, and selenium – and more omega-3 fatty acids, which are essential for brain development and are a protective anti-inflammatory

▶ consists of less convenience food, which means a lower fat intake and far less salt.

In a nutshell, to replenish and protect your health long term, you should enjoy two glasses of red wine every day, at least four portions of vegetables, three of fruit, five to eight servings of good, starchy food like bread, rice, pasta, potatoes, or beans, a small portion of meat, fish, poultry, eggs, and cheese, and modest quantities of olive, canola, or safflower oils.

But don't be a fanatic – a little splurge occasionally really does do you good.

seven-day replenishing

Now you come to the replenishing part of the program. What follows is a week of rainbow eating – lots of brightly colored fruits, vegetables, and salads, all loaded with anti-oxidants. This is what your body needs to give an enormous boost to its natural protective mechanisms.

This is not a rigid regime. You now have some freedom of choice, but do choose as wide a variety of dishes as possible and don't just stick to the ones you like or which are quicker and easier to prepare. The golden rule, though, is that you must eat breakfast, one light meal, and one main meal every day. This is to ensure that you get a wide spread of the essential vitamins, minerals, and trace elements.

the anti-oxidants

Conventional desserts are off the menu. Instead finish every meal with a generous portion of fresh or cooked fruit. Fruits with the highest anti-oxidant value are blueberries, blackberries, blackcurrants, redcurrants, cranberries, strawberries, raspberries, cherries, prunes, raisins, dates, figs, dried apricots, kiwi, black grapes, mango, papaya, passion fruit, citrus fruits, bananas, apples, and pears. You need to eat around 1 pound in weight daily of as wide a mixture of these as you can – and that's a minimum. In fact, at least 1 pound, 10 ounces of what you eat should consist of fruit, vegetables, and salads, and around half your calories should come from the complex carbohydrates – bread, pasta, rice, beans, and so on.

A certain amount of frozen fruit is acceptable as the only serious nutrient loss will be some of the vitamin C, and this is adequately provided elsewhere. But please don't use canned fruits or imagine that the fruits you get in ready-made pies and desserts will be nearly as good.

If you're a vegetarian, don't overdo the eggs and cheese, and if you're a carnivore you'll be enjoying meat, fish, and poultry – but in modest amounts. It's most important to eat three meals a day and you must understand that if you are on any sort of weight loss program, once your calories drop below 1500 a day, it's difficult to get all the nutrients you need to sustain good health (see pages 42–45).

the anti-nutrients

During this week you need to avoid the anti-nutrients – those foods that sap your health and vitality. So this means no takeout, burgers, fries, bags of chips, or high-fat high-sugar cakes, cookies, and pastries. And it's no to instant noodles, soup in a cup and frozen burritos – unless you make your own. In fact, you should eat as little ready-made convenience food as you can possibly manage.

added extras

This week will help make good your nutritional deficiencies. Some nutrients, like minerals and the fat-soluble vitamins A, D and E, can be stored by the body, but others need replenishing daily. So continue to take the multi-vitamin and mineral tablet, as well as the zinc and the probiotic that you were taking during the Cleansing for Health program and now also take the following daily supplements. Continue with them all through the Rebuilding for Health program and for at least a month after that.

- A one-a-day tablet of selenium with vitamins A, C and E
- 500mg fish oil
- A carotenoid supplement that includes lycopene, lutein, and betacarotene
- BioStrath Elixir – the Swiss herbal medicine that boosts natural immunity. Take 1 teaspoon three times a day.

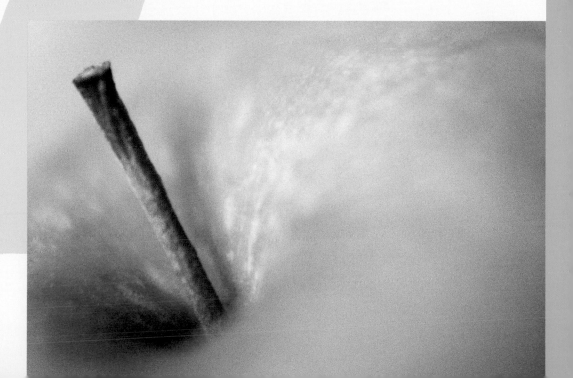

breakfast options

▶ Poached Egg and Tomato (see recipe, page 177) with pink grapefruit juice

▶ Poached Haddock with Cherry Tomatoes (see recipe, page 178) with tomato juice

▶ Kedgeree (see recipe, page 178) with Grape, Pear, Apple, and Pineapple Juice (see recipe, page 189)

▶ Dutch Breakfast (see recipe, page 177) with orange juice

▶ Porridge Muesli (see recipe, page 176) with Apple, Kiwi, Pear, and Celery Juice (see recipe, page 189)

▶ Any whole-wheat cereal with added blueberries, raspberries, or strawberries, and sliced banana, and with Kiwi and Pineapple Juice (see recipe, page 188)

▶ Tomato and Mushroom Omelette (see recipe, page 179) with Yogurt and Prune Smoothie (see recipe, page 189)

light meal options

Three whole-wheat bread or pita pocket sandwiches containing:

▶ A mixture of watercress, grated carrot, spicy sprouts, and chopped, semi-dried apricots mixed with live natural yogurt, black pepper, and a pinch of cayenne; Home-made Chicken Liver Paté (see recipe, page 192) with beansprouts, thinly sliced cucumber, and cranberry sauce; or banana sprinkled with lemon juice to stop it going brown, chopped ready-to-eat prunes, dried cranberries, and peanut butter

▶ Chicken Soup with Barley (see recipe, page 230)

▶ Borscht (see recipe, page 230)

▶ Thick Bean and Barley Soup (see recipe, page 231)

▶ White Soup (see recipe, page 231)

▶ Fruit Crudités with Ricotta Cheese Dip (see recipe, page 238)

▶ Baked Leeks with Cheese and Eggs (see recipe, page 197)

▶ Falafel (see recipe, page 198)

main meal options

▶ Grilled Chicken Breast on Iceberg Lettuce (see recipe, page 193) with rice and mixed vegetables

▶ Baked Stuffed Trout (see recipe, page 195) with Ratatouille (see recipe, page 194)

▶ Stir-Fried Tofu with Vegetables and Noodles (see recipe, page 196)

▶ Game Hen Casserole with Red Cabbage (see recipe, page 198)

▶ Grilled Salmon Steak (see recipe, page 197) with new potatoes, green beans and purple sprouting broccoli

▶ Couscous with Vegetables (see recipe, page 199) with minted yogurt

▶ Organic Beef Stew with Vegetables (see recipe, page 199) with lots of olive-oil mashed potatoes (made with olive oil – no butter, no milk)

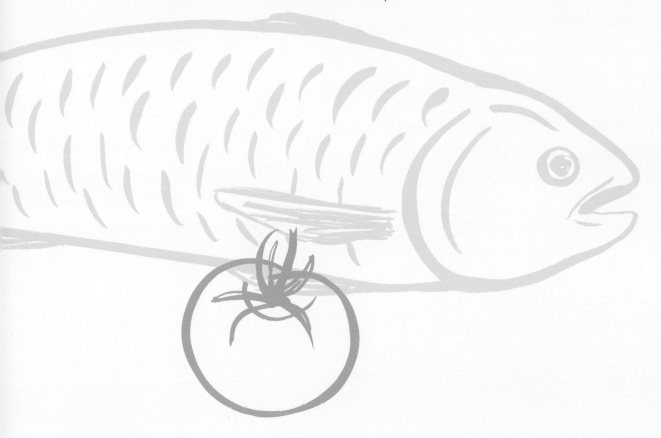

rebuilding for

Now you're into the home strech and you can see the finish line ahead. Over the next two weeks you'll see that time and effort spent preparing and eating good food will repay itself a hundredfold in terms of your health. Unfortunately, even in the best of worlds, other things can interfere with your good intentions. What few people, even doctors, understand is that some prescribed drugs, and even medicines bought over the counter, can have damaging effects on vitamins and minerals. So if you're taking any of the following, you may need more of some foods or supplements to counteract the losses.

antacids

These interfere with vitamins A, B complex, and E, and the minerals calcium, magnesium, iron, and phosphorus. Antacids containing aluminum also reduce the body's absorption of vitamin D.

antibiotics

These destroy the natural bacteria in the gut that manufacture the B vitamins. Neomycin specifically reduces the amount of B12 your body can absorb.

anti-coagulants

These include warfarin and aspirin and affect vitamin K. They are prescribed to prevent clotting so do not take extra doses of vitamin K as this will reduce their effectiveness. They can also reduce absorption of vitamin D.

anti-convulsants

These interfere with vitamins B6, D, and K, and with folic acid. They're normally taken long term, for example in the treatment of epilepsy. Phenytoin (also used to treat irregular heartbeats) interferes with the absorption of calcium.

health

anti-inflammatories

These are often used for the treatment of bowel disease and may cause a loss of folic acid.

anti-ulcer drugs

These work by reducing stomach acid, but can cause poor absorption of B12.

cholesterol-lowering drugs

When used for several months continuously, these can cause poor absorption of iron, betacarotene, vitamins A, D and K, and folic acid.

diuretics

Many of these drugs deprive the body of vitamin B complex, potassium, magnesium, and zinc. Those containing slow-release potassium may have a particularly bad effect on your B12 levels.

laxatives

Regular use lowers the body's levels of calcium, iron and vitamins A, D, and E. Laxative abuse can cause malnutrition and may seriously increase the risk of osteoporosis in later life.

the pill

This has an adverse effect on folic acid, and on vitamins C, E, and B complex.

antidepressants and tranquilizers

These interfere with the absorption of vitamin B2 and with the uptake of zinc and magnesium. Chronic fatigue may be caused by zinc deficiency, yet patients are often prescribed anti-depressants, which lower their zinc levels even more.

fourteen-day rebuilding

For the next two weeks you start by repeating the seven-day Replenishing for Health program. As I'm sure you'll remember – you have done it haven't you? – it isn't an exact eating plan but a chance to choose from a selection of health-replenishing recipes. You also need to keep going with the supplements. I know that the supplement regime may seem like a lot of pills, but it's only for another few weeks, after which you'll have rebuilt your body stores and will only need to take supplements as circumstances dictate.

After the seven-day replenishing plan, you're back to an exact combination of foods for each day of the week. It's fine if you want to switch whole days around or to have the light meals and main meals at whichever time of day suits you best. But what you mustn't do is to take a light meal from one day, a main meal from another and breakfast from a third, as this will not achieve the ideal balance.

For the whole two weeks, don't exceed 14 drinks of alcohol a week if you're a woman, 21 for a man, and don't drink more than a total of four cups of tea and coffee on any one day. Canned fizzy drinks are still taboo but you can drink as much herb tea, fresh unsweetened fruit juice or salt-free vegetable juice as you like. Of course you still need at least one and a half quarts of water a day.

Days 1–7, follow the Seven-Day Replenishing program.

day 8

breakfast
Any hot cereal with a sprinkle of raisins, honey, and cinnamon

Kiwi and Pineapple Juice (see recipe, page 188)

light meal
Special Welsh Rarebit (see recipe, page 194)

Spinach with Yogurt (see recipe, page 199)

A pear with a small piece of soft cheese (preferably goat's) and a bunch of red grapes

main meal
Grilled Marinated Fish (see recipe, page 200) with Mixed Cabbage, Leek, and Green Onions, (see recipe, page 200) and olive-oil mashed potatoes (made with olive oil – no butter, no milk)

Yogurt and Mango Smoothie (see recipe, page 188)

day 9

breakfast
Poached Haddock with Cherry Tomatoes (see recipe, page 178)

2 thin slices of unbuttered whole-wheat bread

Apple, Kiwi, Pear, and Celery juice (see recipe, page 189)

light meal
Onion Soup (see recipe, page 236) with a chunk of whole-wheat bread

Salad made from half a sliced avocado, dark green lettuce and tomato and watercress, sprinkled with toasted sunflower seeds

A pear

main meal
Chicken Jalfrezi (see recipe, page 201)

Carrot Salad (see recipe, page 238)

2 pieces of fresh fruit – not bananas

day 10

breakfast   Dutch Breakfast (see recipe, page 177)

Grape, Pear, Apple, and Pineapple Juice (see recipe, page 189)

light meal   Creamy Mackerel with Eggs (see recipe, page 219)

Watercress Salad (see recipe, page 237)

Stewed apple with live natural yogurt

main meal   Grilled Lamb Chops with Rosemary (see recipe, page 210), Bulgur with Eggplant (see recipe, page 202) and a mixed green salad

Fresh pineapple

day 11

breakfast   Zucchini and Cheddar Omelette (see recipe, page 179)

Tomato Juice, Celery, and Celery Leaf Blend (see recipe, page 188)

light meal   Pasta Noodles with Broccoli (see recipe, page 202) with a tomato and onion salad

Wholemilk yogurt with a teaspoon of honey, sprinkled with chopped hazelnuts

main meal   Salmon in a Parcel (see recipe, page 203) with mixed green salad

Strawberries, raspberries, blueberries, and a little light cream

day 12

breakfast   Sautéed Wild Mushrooms and Walnuts (see recipe, page 179) on whole-wheat toast

Carrot, Apple, and Celery juice (see recipe, page 187)

light meal   Deviled Sardines (see recipe, page 194) with whole-wheat pita bread and a salad of avocado and watercress sprinkled with pine nuts

2 plums

main meal   Crudités with French dressing

Grilled Paprika Chicken (see recipe, page 221) with brown rice drizzled with olive oil and some finely chopped garlic

A small piece of hard cheese and an apple

day 13

breakfast   Fresh Fruit Kebabs (see recipe, page 177)
Berry Smoothie (see recipe, page 189)

light meal   Oat and Broccoli Soup (see recipe, page 236) with a chunk of dark rye or mixed-grain bread
A mixed green salad
A piece of soft cheese, preferably goat's, with an apple

main meal   Pan-Fried Liver (see recipe, page 203) with cauliflower, broccoli, and new potatoes
A thinly sliced banana, with honey and a little light cream, sprinkled with toasted sunflower seeds

day 14

breakfast   Porridge Muesli (see recipe, page 176)
Orange Juice and Almond Blend (see recipe, page 188)

light meal   Scrambled eggs on a bed of puréed spinach sprinkled with nutmeg
A small piece of strong Cheddar cheese and 2 stalks of celery (with leaves)

main meal   Braised Chicken (see recipe, page 226) with spring greens, dark cabbage or kale, carrots, and plain boiled potatoes
A generous bowl of any berries with sour cream or mascarpone cheese

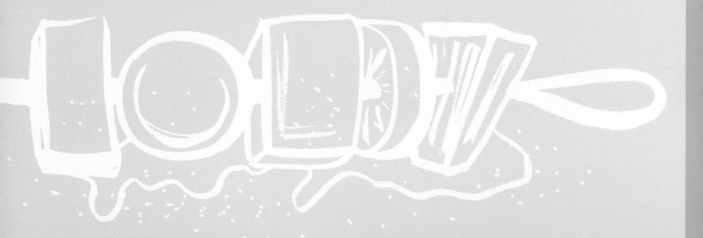

healthy eating

The first path to super health is healthy eating. "You are what you eat" says the proverb, and of course it's true. But unfortunately, what most people don't realize is that you're also what you don't eat. In spite of the mountain of information out there about health and its relationship to nutrition, food, and cooking, the messages get confused. As a result, I see in my office an ever-increasing number of people who are either overfed yet undernourished, or so busy trying to follow every piece of food advice they read or hear that they end up underfed and, of course, undernourished.

It's extraordinary that with the never-ending stream of cookbooks that are published, the seemingly limitless number of TV shows about food, the huge amount of newspaper and magazine coverage of this topic, and the hundreds of websites devoted to food, health, and nutrition, the average shopper still gets it wrong and seems unable to make sensible choices.

But how do you choose when there are so many conflicting messages? Don't eat eggs – eat eggs; eat margarine – eat butter; eat soy products – don't eat soy products; you need salt – you don't need salt; skim milk is healthy – full-fat milk is healthy; chocolate is good – chocolate is bad; eat meat – be a vegetarian. . . . No wonder everyone's confused and alarmed by each new report that makes the headlines.

It's enough to make you wonder how our great-grandparents and grandparents ever survived in the 1920s and 1930s without the army of dietitians, nutritionists (qualified and bogus), holistic health experts, and lifestyle coaches that exist today. In fact, in many ways their lives were better than ours. There was less obesity, less heart disease, less cancer – and eating disorders were virtually unknown. People only ate food that was in season and mothers relied on their common sense and on the skills they'd learned from their mothers to raise healthy, well-fed families. It's just as easy to do this today. Thanks to the enormous variety of food available, it only takes a little thought to make sure you and your family get an abundance of all the essential nutrients, yet avoid the excesses that cause disease.

the three-box trick

Next time you go shopping, put three equal-size boxes in your supermarket cart and follow these easy rules for your one-week family food supply.

The first box should be filled to the brim with good quality carbohydrates – potatoes, rice, pasta, bread, beans, oatmeal, granola, whole-grain breakfast cereals, and whole-wheat flakes. The second box must overflow with fruit, and vegetables. You should also include dried fruits, fresh nuts, and seeds. Frozen vegetables are fine if they suit your lifestyle better; they are almost as nutritious as fresh vegetables. The third box is a little more complicated. Just imagine it's divided into three compartments – two of equal-size that together take up 80 per cent of the space and a third occupying the last 20 per cent. The first of the two equal-size compartments contains your cheese, milk, yogurt and eggs. The second is filled with purchases of meat, fish, and poultry or with vegetarian protein such as tofu, or textured vegetable protein (TVP), and the final tiny space is the one where you put the cream, cookies, sweets, chocolates, sweet rolls, and other treats.

Use exactly the same proportions as the basis of your daily diet when you get home. That way you'll get at least half your calories from good carbohydrates, no more than a third of them from fat, and between 10 and 12 per cent of them from protein. And by adding a couple of glasses of wine a day, your calories from alcohol will be less than 10 per cent of your daily calorie intake and won't exceed the recommended maximum number of drinks.

how to gain weight & build beautiful muscles

If you're desperate to put on some weight and rebuild your health, surprisingly, the best starting point is exercise. Not aerobics, jogging, or marathon running, but real old-fashioned weight training and body building. This will build bigger muscles and dramatically improve your body shape, but it must go together with a dramatic increase in your good calorie consumption. What you must not do is to get these extra calories from high-sugar, high-fat foods that will make you gain weight but will dramatically increase your risk of a heart attack at the same time.

good calories

The healthiest calories come from complex carbohydrates like whole-grain bread, oats, potatoes, pasta, rice, and beans. They should make up at least half of your daily food, but there is a limit to how much you can eat at one time. Get extra calories from bananas, unsalted nuts, and dried fruits. Raisins, dates, and dried apricots are excellent sources of vitamins, minerals, and fiber, and eaten as snacks, they add a significant number of calories in a comparatively small amount of food.

Other sources of healthy calories are seeds. Sunflower and sesame seeds are especially good, and peanut butter and tahini — a spread made from crushed sesame — provide a large number of calories, plenty of essential rebuilding nutrients, and very little bulk.

grazing's ok

This is the time for you to become a grazer — aim to eat something at least every two hours, starting with a really good breakfast and finishing with a bedtime snack. Dips like guacamole, made from avocado and olive oil, or hummus, made with chickpeas and tahini, eaten with whole-wheat pita bread, make excellent between-meal snacks and, like all the best foods, provide a high proportion of nutrients with their calories.

the healthy weight gain secret weapon

For all of you who suffer severe embarrassment through being underweight, here's the secret weapon in my Healthy Weight Gain Plan. It's a recipe that I've used successfully for years in my own practice. It's also excellent for anyone undergoing chemotherapy who may not feel like or be able to eat "proper" food. Make it up first thing in the morning, drink a glass of it before breakfast, keep the rest in the fridge and make sure it's all gone by bedtime.

You'll need 2 cups of whole milk, one certified salmonella-free raw egg, one banana, 2 teaspoons each of molasses, honey, tahini, wheatgerm, and brewer's yeast powder, and four dried apricots. Mix all the ingredients together in a blender and enjoy.

down with obesity

The US National Center for Health Statistics reports that a third of American adults are so overweight that they exceed the maximum safe Body Mass Index. And judged by World Health Organization standards, almost 60 per cent of men and 50 per cent of women in America would be considered at risk through being overweight or obese. In addition, the US government now calculates that illness caused by obesity — high blood pressure, strokes, heart disease, gallstones, diabetes, cancer, arthritis — costs an annual $66 billion.

Throughout the world the picture is similar and, most alarmingly, it's the rate at which obesity has increased in children that will set the pattern for a pandemic of weight-related illnesses in the coming years. In the last 25 years in the USA, the number of obese youngsters has more than tripled. Frighteningly, this effect is apparent in virtually all ethnic groups and at every socio-economic level. Even in Egypt there are nearly four times as many seriously fat children as there were 18 years ago. One worrying result of this is the growing epidemic of adult-onset or Type II diabetes — often called Non-Insulin Dependent Diabetes. This illness has always been regarded as something likely to happen in a person's late forties or fifties, but it's now showing up in children as young as eight.

Why are so many people now overweight? Although many people today consume 800 calories a day less than they did in the 1950s, we're eating 50 per cent more fat and almost everyone, including children, is far less physically active, both at work and leisure. And while the diet industry pushes the lose-weight message, the multinational food industry encourages an ever-increasing consumption of high-fat, high-sugar convenience and junk foods.

I'm afraid there are no magic answers to being overweight, and after almost 40 years in practice I've probably heard all the excuses — big bones, slow metabolism, glandular problems, hormone imbalance, thyroid disorders, genetic influences, and the "I hardly eat a thing so I don't know why I'm gaining weight" syndrome. Of course there are medical conditions and certain prescribed drugs which can cause weight gain and make losing weight extremely hard, but these are comparatively rare. For 90 per cent of the

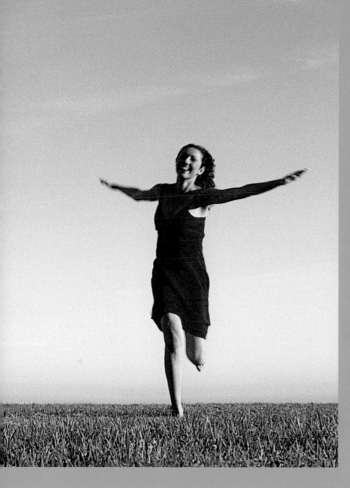

people who are overweight, the answer is extremely simple. If you consume more calories than you burn, your weight goes up, and if you burn more calories than you consume, it goes down.

Here are three simple suggestions that I promise you work.

▶ If you eat two slices of bread and butter a day less and walk 15 minutes a day more, you'll lose a pound a week without doing anything else.

▶ If you stand up whenever you speak on the telephone, you'll lose over four pounds a year – it takes more muscle effort to stand than to sit.

▶ And if you use a remote control for your TV, you'll gain two pounds a year.

There are no miracle diets, though it's true there are some that make you lose weight quickly. Unfortunately, they're either unhealthy, unsustainable or both, and the minute you stop dieting you put back on all the weight you've lost, plus a pound or two. And each time you do that, your fat deposits move further up your body, so you gradually change from a healthy pear shape to an unhealthy apple shape – the more fat you carry around your middle, the greater the risk of heart disease.

Forget the cabbage-soup diet – it's anti-social. Forget high-protein diets – they can seriously damage your kidneys. And forget eating for your blood group, eating nothing but fruit before lunch and any other cranky diet idea that flies in the face of normal balanced eating. All you have to do to keep your weight under control is to eat good healthy food on a regular basis.

And just remember, it's what you eat most of the time that counts – what you eat occasionally doesn't matter a bit.

the ten-day weight loss plan

This ten-day eating plan is not only balanced and healthy, providing you with an excellent spread of essential nutrients, but will also help you achieve a sensible and sustainable weight loss. You can repeat the plan as many times as you like, and if you're overweight you'll lose one to two pounds a week. You may be surprised at how much food you'll be eating every day, but don't skip any of the meals – each one is there for a purpose. It's fine to switch the days around or to switch meals on each day, but this plan works best if you don't mix and match meals from different days.

There's no calorie counting, no weighing of portions. All I ask is that you use your common sense and don't go overboard when it comes to butter and oils. And you mustn't miss out on the starchy foods like pasta, rice, potatoes, and bread, as these provide vital fiber, vitamins and minerals, as well as the calories needed to stimulate your metabolism and provide you with energy. This is one weight-loss plan that won't leave you feeling tired, hungry, depressed, and irritable.

every day
Start every day with a large glass of hot water with the juice of half a lime – no sugar. Always eat the breakfast, and it's a good idea to take a one-a-day multi-vitamin and mineral supplement. Some people find it easier to eat less at a time, but more frequently. That's no problem; save some of the foods from each meal and use them as mid-morning, afternoon, and late night snacks. That way you eat all the day's meals and you won't snack on forbidden "extras."

Drink at least one and a half quarts of fluid a day, a liter of which should be water. Two cups of real coffee and two cups of tea with milk but no sugar are OK, but for other hot drinks, stick to herbal teas without milk. Although small amounts of alcohol are generally good for the health, I would advise against drinking any during this first ten days. If you decide to repeat the plan, then a couple of glasses of wine, a couple of beers, or two shots of spirits twice a week are fine.

day 1

breakfast   A whole pink grapefruit and 2 slices of whole-wheat toast with a very thin scraping of butter and honey

light meal   Avocado, Tomato, and Mushroom Salad (see recipe, page 240)

main meal   Borscht (see recipe, page 230)
Grilled Chicken Breast on Iceberg lettuce (see recipe, page 193) with corn, fava beans, and boiled potatoes
Fresh fruit

day 2

breakfast   Poached Egg and Tomato (see recipe, page 177) and 1 slice of whole-wheat toast with a thin scraping of butter

light meal   Vegetable Soup (see recipe, page 229) and 1 whole-wheat roll – no butter

main meal   Grilled Marinated Fish (see recipe, page 200) with spinach and rice
A selection of dried fruits

day 3

breakfast   A large glass of orange juice
Porridge Muesli (see recipe, page 176)

light meal   Pasta Noodles with Broccoli (see recipe, page 202)
Celery Salad (see recipe, page 238)

main meal   Mixed Vegetable Stir-Fry with Rice (see recipe, page 192)
A sliced banana and live natural yogurt, sprinkled with sesame seeds

day 4

breakfast   Dutch Breakfast (see recipe, page 177)

light meal   Lettuce Soup (see recipe, page 229), 1 whole-wheat roll, no butter
Selection of fresh fruit – not bananas

main meal   Grilled Lamb Chops with Rosemary (see recipe, page 210)
Mixed Cabbage, Leek, and Green Onions (see recipe, page 200)
A fresh fruit salad of mango, kiwi, and pineapple

day 5

breakfast   A large bowl of any hot cereal made with half-water, half-milk, and sprinkled with
raisins, honey, and cinnamon; 1 slice of whole-wheat toast with a thin scraping of butter
A large glass of orange juice

light meal   Grapefruit, Peach, and Mascarpone Salad (see recipe, page 239) and 2 rye crispbreads
with a thin scraping of butter

main meal   Couscous with Vegetables (see recipe, page 199)
Fresh Fruit Kebabs (see recipe, page 177)

day 6

breakfast   Yogurt and Prune Smoothie (see recipe, page 189), 1 thick slice of whole-wheat toast
with a thin scraping of butter, a ripe banana

light meal   Tomato and Mushroom Omelette (see recipe, page 179) with a green salad

main meal   Organic Beef Stew with Vegetables (see recipe, page 199)
Natural live yogurt with a teaspoon of honey and a generous sprinkling of toasted pine nuts

day 7

breakfast   Kiwi and Pineapple Juice (see recipe, page 188)
Natural live yogurt with a sliced banana, fresh blueberries, and honey

light meal   Tuna and Cottage-Cheese Stuffed Tomatoes (see recipe, page 196) with new potatoes

main meal   Bulgur with Eggplant (see recipe, page 202)
Cucumber and Strawberry Salad (see recipe, page 237)
An apple, a pear, and a matchbox-size piece of your favorite cheese

day 8
breakfast   Tomato Juice, Celery, and Celery Leaf Blend (see recipe, page 188)
A bowl of any good quality unsweetened muesli

light meal   Watercress Salad (see recipe, page 237), 4 canned sardines in olive oil
2 slices of whole-wheat toast with a thin scraping of butter

main meal   Grilled Paprika Chicken (see recipe, page 221) with Tsatsiki (see recipe, page 238), rice and green beans
An orange and a bunch of grapes

day 9
breakfast   Berry Smoothie (see recipe, page 189)
2 slices of whole-wheat toast with thinly sliced cheese and tomato – no butter

light meal   Pasta with Lettuce Pesto (see recipe, page 193)
A small bunch of grapes and a kiwi fruit

main meal   Pan-Fried Liver (see recipe, page 203) with mashed potatoes made with olive oil instead of
butter, shredded cooked cabbage and Carrot Salad (see recipe, page 238)
An apple, a pear, and a few grapes

day 10
breakfast   Orange Juice and Almond Blend (see recipe, page 188), a banana, an apple, and some grapes

light meal   Falafel (see recipe, page 198) with Tomato, Red Onion, and Beet Salad (see recipe, page
239), a mango

main meal   Oat and Broccoli Soup (see recipe, page 236)
Salmon in a Parcel (see recipe, page 203) with new potatoes and Watercress Salad (see
recipe, page 237)
A mixture of dried fruits and unsalted nuts

staying active

Staying active is the second path to super health. The best diet in the world won't help you stay healthy if you can't get up the stairs, walk to the store, or cut the grass. So if you want permanent good health, you have to exercise and keep active. This doesn't mean putting on a leotard, buying expensive running shoes, and sweating in a gym, nor does physical activity have to be confined to the young and beautiful. Whether you're 8 or 80, getting your body moving through regular exercise results in dramatic improvements in the way it functions.

Exercise builds muscle strength, which improves posture, prevents backache, and reduces the pain of arthritis. It specifically improves the health and efficiency of lungs, circulation, and the heart. And as your heart grows stronger it's able to pump more blood with fewer beats and less effort, which reduces the strain on the heart itself and prolongs its healthy active life.

Regular exercise also boosts your natural immunity and increases the body's resistance to disease and infection. It also makes you feel good emotionally, as physical activity releases mood-boosting hormones in the brain. The most important thing is to choose an activity you enjoy and one that's appropriate to your age, ability, and general health. It doesn't matter if it's walking the dog, bowling, windsurfing, or riding a bike – half an hour, three times a week will improve your health permanently.

And remember, most fashionable exercise regimes are fine if you're fit, but are definitely not a good place to start if you're not. And if you're thinking of a personal trainer, check that they're properly qualified and know what they're doing.

are you fit to exercise?

Before starting any exercise program you must assess your own fitness. If you are overweight and over 40 and you've hardly moved a muscle since you left school, seek professional advice before you start. And the same is true if you've ever been told that you have high blood pressure or heart disease. To help you decide how you stand, answer the following questions **truthfully**, then add up the number of yeses.

1   Are you over 40?

2   Is it more than 5 years since you took regular exercise?

3   Do you regularly get home and fall asleep in front of the TV?

4   Do you have any joint disease or deformity?

5   Are you more than 15 pounds overweight?

6   Do you ever get dizzy or faint?

7   Do you smoke?

8   Do you feel ill if you have had to run for any reason?

9   Do you get out of breath easily?

10 Do you have a problem sleeping?

11 Have you ever had a serious back problem?

12 Do you drink more than four 12-ounce beers, 3 glasses of wine or 3 spirits daily?

0–3 yeses   Good, but start exercising today

3–6 yeses   Just in time; start gently and persevere

6–12 yeses You may not make it to the gym! Get some advice before you start.

getting mobile

Fitness is a combination of strength, mobility, and stamina and ideally you need all three. There's no point in being strong if you can't bend down to tie your shoelace, or extremely mobile if you can't keep up with your children on a 2-mile walk.

Staying mobile also helps you to maintain your youth and vitality. I have many patients in their eighties and nineties whom I could easily take for being twenty or thirty years younger when I see them walk effortlessly into the consulting room, get themselves easily onto the treatment table or bend smoothly to pick something up from the floor.

And if you suffer from any arthritic problems, maintaining and improving your mobility is even more vital. The stiffer the affected joints become, the more painful they get and the less you can use them, which leads you into a downward spiral. There are now many studies that prove conclusively that arthritis is not a reason for inactivity. The more you exercise the joints, the more you improve your mobility, strengthen the supportive muscles, and reduce the pain.

my top three exercises for mobility

▶ A good starting point for improving mobility is yoga. If you haven't exercised for a while, yoga's a safe way to start gently stretching and mobilizing your joints, muscles, and ligaments without the risk of injury. Yoga also provides the added bonus of improved breath control and mental as well as physical relaxation. The concentration required helps eliminate stress and anxiety, so reducing the levels of adrenaline circulating in the bloodstream. This helps to lower blood pressure and reduce the strain on the heart and blood vessels.

▶ Swimming is another excellent activity and is ideal if you spend most of your working life at a desk or in front of a computer, where poor posture maintained for long periods at a time results in a shortening of muscles, tendons, and ligaments and a gradual loss of joint mobility. When you're swimming, 70 per cent of your bodyweight is supported by the water so you'll find that stiff hips and knees, rigid backs and immobile neck and shoulder joints all move far more easily when they are free from the strains of weightbearing. An added bonus is that swimming can substantially improve your breathing, so it's a particularly valuable form of exercise for asthmatics.

▶ You can combine straightforward swimming with aquarobics – specially designed exercises to do in the pool. Initially it's best to learn these in a class. Once you've mastered them, you can combine them with your regular swimming sessions.

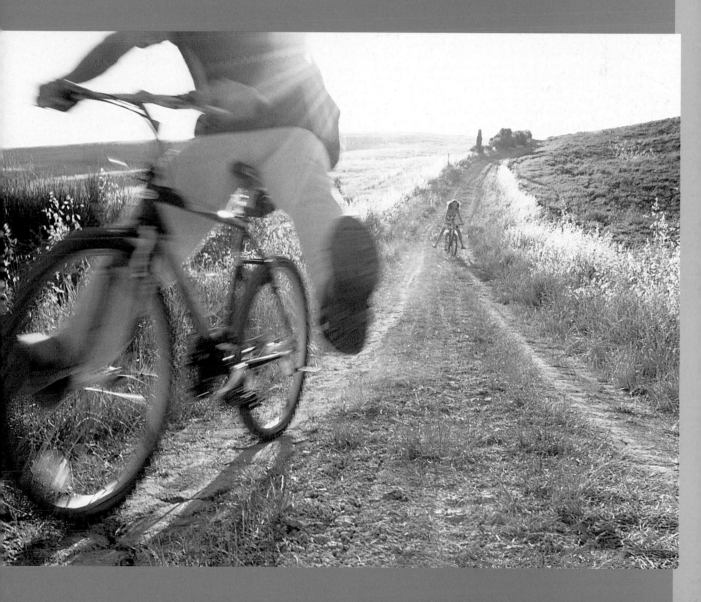

building and maintaining stamina

Once you've gotten mobile, building and maintaining stamina is the next step. This can only be achieved by increasing the working efficiency of your heart, circulation, and lungs and by developing greater muscle strength. You do this by gradually increasing the workload of your exercise regime and extending the length of time for which you keep up the activity.

Always precede your exercises with a sequence of warm-ups, and end with a cool-down sequence. The warm-ups will gently stretch the muscles, speed up the circulation, and increase your pulse rate. They also start the release of the body's feel-good hormones that put you in the right frame of mind for the exercise to follow. Your warm-up should last a minimum of five minutes and it's just as important if you're a regular athlete as it is if you're starting from scratch.

The endurance stage of your program should last for 20–30 minutes, during which you push your heart rate up to the appropriate level (see table opposite) and keep it there. You shouldn't end up gasping for breath but as your stamina increases, you'll need to increase the length of exercise or its intensity. In the early stages, it's better to exercise less vigorously but for slightly longer periods.

The cooling-down phase is vital as it allows your heart rate and breathing to return to normal gradually, while the combination of stretching and alternate walking and jogging lets your muscles cool down slowly. You need at least six minutes in this phase.

Whatever you do, remember that your exercise regime should be fun and you mustn't allow it to become an obsession. You may find you prefer to stick to one activity, like tennis, though you'll get a better balance of strength and mobility if you do a range of different sports. A session in the gym, a session of your favorite sport, and a swim is a great weekly combination. With a bit of experimentation you'll soon find what fits best with your personal preferences, work, and lifestyle.

a word of warning

Great though it is to increase your activity, do not exercise if

▶ you have a heavy cold or a raised temperature

▶ you have or develop pain in the chest

▶ you have persistent joint or muscle pains for which you haven't had professional advice

▶ the weather is extremely hot or extremely cold

top tips for safe activity

Check your heart rate. Most adult men and women have a resting heart rate of 60–80 beats per minute. Find yours by pressing your wrist on the thumb side, counting the beats for 15 seconds, then multiplying by four to find the rate per minute. When you exercise, you should aim to push your heart rate up to the level recommended below.

▶ When warming up and cooling down, make sure you do the stretching exercises slowly and gradually. Any short jerky movements will make your muscles contract and be more liable to damage.

▶ Don't worry if you feel a bit stiff to begin with. Your body simply isn't accustomed to exercise. These aches and pains will stop as you get fitter.

▶ Keeping well hydrated is extremely important, but stick to plain water and avoid fizzy drinks as these can make you bloated and uncomfortable. Unless you're working extremely hard, you have no need whatsoever of sports drinks or energy boosters. A banana or some dried fruits an hour before you exercise, plenty of water during your activity, and more water or diluted orange juice afterwards is adequate.

▶ Remember that you're trying to train not strain, so build up your exercise gradually. One of the major risks is being too competitive and though there are people for whom winning is important, when you're building up your activity levels is not the time. Trying to keep up with a friend who's been doing aerobics classes for years or challenging the new office junior to a game of squash when you haven't played for 20 years are both recipes for disaster.

▶ Take a shower or bath to cool down and relax your tired muscles after exercise. Take your time, don't rush, and enjoy it. This is a reward for you and your muscles.

▶ I've learned from experience with my patients that it's far more effective to do your fitness routine with a partner. It's a lot more fun and if you know someone is waiting for you at the gym, the park, or the swimming pool, you're more likely to keep going.

age	beats per min
20	138–158
25	137–156
30	135–154
35	134–153
40	132–151
45	131–150
50	129–147
55	127–146
60	126–144
65	125–142
70	123–141
75	122–139
80	120–138
85	119–136

mental attitude

The third path to a healthy life is having a positive mental attitude. You can't separate the mind from the body and I've seen the effects of this relationship many times, in both my professional and my private life. Way back in the late 1950s, when I was a student, I worked as a lowly orderly in one of the world's pioneering spinal injuries centers at Stoke Mandeville Hospital near Aylesbury in Buckinghamshire.

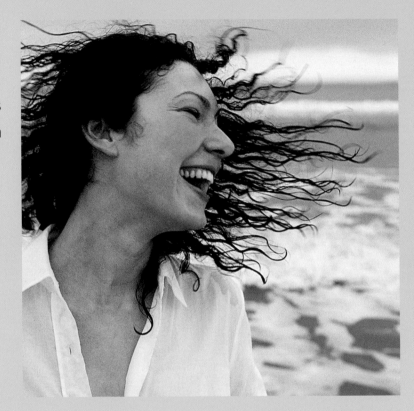

I soon learned the power of positive thought when I was looking after two young men, both paralyzed from the chest down and both with identical degrees of disability. One was a soldier who'd been shot in the back, the other an affluent lawyer who'd fallen off his horse. The soldier's family was poor and lived far away, so he was on his own. The lawyer's family was rich, rented a house to be near the hospital, paid for a private room, and smothered the lawyer with love and support. The soldier was desperate to be independent and was soon able to get himself off the bed, into a wheelchair and take part in the rough and tumble of wheelchair basketball. The lawyer simply turned his face to the wall and died. As it turned out, the only real difference between them was their attitude to their problem.

happiness fights disease

There's long been a suspicion that positive, happy people with a sense of inner peace are healthier than negative ones. A South African doctor once wrote a book called "Happy People Don't Get Cancer" – a sweeping and not wholly accurate generalization. But it is certain that happy, positive people tend to have a stronger natural resistance to all sorts of disease. And as my story of the paralyzed men shows, this happiness has little to do with material wealth.

Research at the University of Cleveland, Ohio, has now established that the mental attitude of cancer patients can make a profound difference to the outcome of their illness. In their research, patients with a positive mental attitude who saw themselves as survivors rather than victims and who played an active part in their own healing process fared the best.

Once again, it's thanks to the complex relationship between the mental and the physical. All the evidence now shows that positive people tend to have higher levels of the special white blood cells that attack bacteria and viruses. These white blood cells are the body's first line of immune defense.

So if you're able to enjoy inner peace and happiness, whether it's through your own strength, through strong religious beliefs, or simply part of your personality, you are indeed fortunate. Cultivate it, build on it, and use it, because happiness is the one thing you can give away to other people without depleting your own. In fact, it's just the opposite. Sharing your happiness increases your own supply and helps promote your health to even higher levels.

think positive

Do you see your glass as half full or half empty? Yes, I know it's an old chestnut but, in the words of the comedian, the old ones are the best. The glass question in fact has a serious underlying message. For those who are naturally positive about life, their glass is always half full, not half empty and, as I've already said, positive equates to healthy.

People who see their glass as half empty are often those who find it impossible to take responsibility for their own actions. They believe the grass is always greener on the other side of the fence and think it's always someone else's fault they didn't get that promotion. They're convinced that the world is against them, and they end up being eaten up by negative thoughts, petty jealousies, and miseries. They're no fun to be with, they're always complaining and blaming and, not surprisingly, they're nearly always ill.

combat negativity

Many sayings that have been around for years – "smile in the face of adversity," "look on the bright side," "keep your chin up" – are actually exhortations to be positive. They have stood the test of time because they actually work.

One of the pioneers in the use of self-help to combat negativity was the French psychotherapist Emile Coué. In the early 1900s he started a free clinic where he treated patients on the basis that learning to use the imagination can bring about self-healing. He encouraged his patients to repeat the now famous mantra "Every day and in every way I am becoming better and better," believing that if this was repeated often enough at times when the mind was most receptive, it would plant positive thoughts deep in the subconscious and these would push out the negative beliefs that were causing the unhappiness and disease.

six simple positivity-boosting exercises

Certain physical exercises can help boost your positivity and so enhance your health. Try some of these.

1 Clasp the fingers of both hands behind your head. Lift your chin and push hard against your hands for 10 seconds. Repeat 5 times.

2 Place your palms against your forehead. Try to push your chin down by pressing your head against your hands. Hold for 10 seconds. Repeat 5 times.

3 Put your left hand against the left side of your head and try to push your left ear towards your left shoulder. At the same time, push your hand against the side of your head. Hold for 10 seconds. Repeat 5 times. Repeat on the right side.

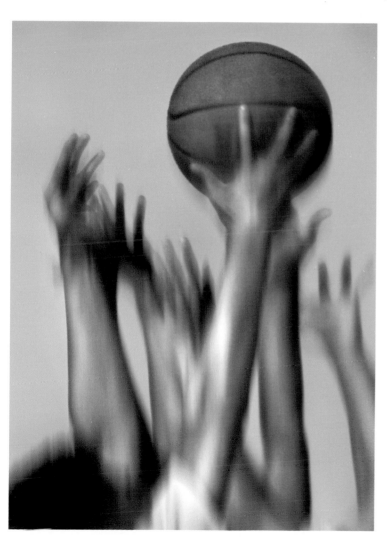

4 Standing or sitting, raise your shoulders as high as you can, with your arms hanging by your sides. Hold for 5 seconds, then let your shoulders drop with their own weight. Repeat 5 times.

5 Standing or sitting, push both shoulders back as far as you can, sticking out your chest and forcing your shoulder blades together. Hold for 5 seconds and relax. Repeat 3 times.

6 Standing or sitting, push both shoulders as far forward as you can, narrowing your chest and forcing your shoulder blades as far apart as they will go, with your arms hanging down. Hold for 5 seconds and relax. Repeat 3 times.

a good night's sleep

Are you surprised to know that a bottle of milk, a spoonful of honey, a loaf of bread, and lettuce are all you need to get a better night's sleep? A glass of warm milk with honey is a time-honored aid to sleep, but have it at bedtime with a lettuce sandwich and you'll be off to the land of nod before you can count ten sheep.

None of us can escape the occasional bad night. Indigestion, toothache, backache, anxiety, being too hot or too cold, a snoring partner . . . these are just some of the things that can conspire to rob us of our beauty sleep.

But real insomnia is a state of habitual sleeplessness repeated night after night, often for months or even years on end. On top of that, worrying about the insomnia, often to the point of obsession, does more damage than the lack of sleep itself. But there's no need to limp through the rest of your life on the crutch of sleeping pills, tranquilizers, or alcohol.

my top tips for a good night's rest

▶ What you eat before bedtime is key. Going to bed too full or too hungry both interfere with sleep, as does eating too late, especially if it's animal protein. This type of food is a mental stimulant and triggers the body to produce more activity hormones. Starchy foods, on the other hand, encourage the body to manufacture more tryptophan, the brain's own calming chemical, and the non-active, growth, and repair hormones. So ideally, evening meals should be based on foods like rice, pasta, potatoes, bread, root vegetables, and beans, and you should save the meat meals for the middle of the day.

▶ Eat a bedtime sandwich. Any sandwich will help, but the best filling is lettuce, a strong soporific. In 1789 one of the great herbalists, Sir John Hill, published his **Family Herbal**. In it he writes about the wild lettuce, used by the ancient Romans as a sleep inducer: "It eases the most violent pain in colics and other disorders and gently disposes the person to sleep. It has the good effect of a gentle opiate, and none of the bad ones of that violent medicine." How right he was.

Eat your herbs. Sage, fennel, rosemary, and basil are all calming, soothing, and sleep-inducing, thanks to the essential oils they contain, so try to include some in your evening meal. Herb teas – especially camomile and linden – can be as effective as many sleeping pills. As well as containing calming chemicals, they are entirely free from caffeine which, for many people, is sleep's greatest enemy.

If your children can't sleep, cut down on their cola intake. I'm always appalled when I see parents allowing young children to consume quantities of cola drinks. They would be horrified if someone offered their eight-year-old a double espresso, but seem to have no qualms about them getting substantial doses of caffeine from the cola. Is it any wonder that so many youngsters have disturbed sleep patterns, feel tired all day at school, fall behind in their learning, and on top of all that develop behavioral difficulties too?

Improve your sleep with aromatherapy oils. They work both when absorbed through the skin or inhaled, so add them to a warm bath, get your partner to give you a gentle aromatherapy massage, sprinkle them on your pillow, or use them in a burner. Lavender is one of the best. A study some years ago revealed that a lavender burner in a ward of elderly patients was as effective as the sleeping pills most of them were taking – but of course the patients didn't suffer any unwanted side effects. A wonderful soporific mixture for the bath is 3 drops of basil oil, 2 drops of orange oil and 5 drops of lavender oil, stirred into a tablespoon of any light cooking oil. For massage use 2 drops each of marjoram, rose, and lavender to 2 tablespoons of oil – grape-seed or almond oils are best for massage.

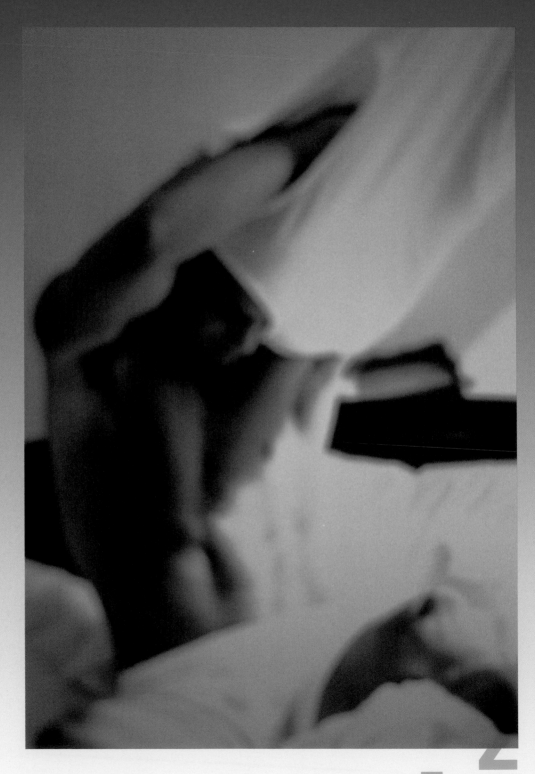

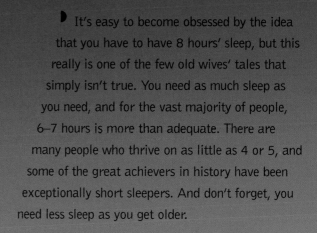

It's easy to become obsessed by the idea that you have to have 8 hours' sleep, but this really is one of the few old wives' tales that simply isn't true. You need as much sleep as you need, and for the vast majority of people, 6–7 hours is more than adequate. There are many people who thrive on as little as 4 or 5, and some of the great achievers in history have been exceptionally short sleepers. And don't forget, you need less sleep as you get older.

Finally, if you really can't sleep, don't just lie there worrying. Get up and do some of the boring chores you need to catch up on – the ironing, writing a shopping list, clearing out the cutlery drawer, paying those unpaid bills. Don't turn on the television and watch the midnight thriller, and don't start reading the latest bestseller or you'll be there till dawn. Do something dull and you'll soon find that bed beckons.

natural aids to a good night's sleep

These herbal remedies are non-addictive, don't disturb your natural sleep patterns, and won't leave you feeling as if you've got a hangover the next morning. Because they're gentler than conventional drugs they don't work instantly and you may need to persevere for a few nights before you get maximum benefit.

Extract of passiflora promotes natural sleep. It's perfect if you get to sleep without any problems but keep waking during the night.

A standardized extract of valerian calms and soothes away the stresses of a hectic life. It's the answer for people who find it hard to get off to sleep.

Linden (tilia) tea with added honey.

leisure = pleasure = health

Believe it or not, in England there's a scientific body called ARISE. Some of their prestigious meetings include lavish dinners where many different wines are served with each course, and the diners eat foie gras, goose, chocolate pudding, cheese, and petits fours. Then they are encouraged to enjoy a large Havana cigar with their port and the meal finishes with strong black coffee.

Appalling? No, because ARISE is an acronym for Associates for Research Into the Science of Enjoyment. Like me, its members are increasingly concerned that the "food and health police" are creating a world where enjoyment and pleasure stand for sin and guilt. We've seen earlier how important a positive attitude is in the creation and preservation of good health, and I can't repeat too often that as far as nutrition is concerned it's what you do most of the time that's important, while what you do occasionally is of little consequence. Little consequence except, that is, when what you do occasionally gives you pleasure. And for the benefit of your health, pleasure should be the object of your leisure time.

The reasons for this are not just psychological. When you're stressed – as so many of us are these days – the constant over-production of adrenaline increases your heart rate, speeds your respiration, and increases your blood pressure. Enjoyable activities counteract all these adverse physiological effects.

In addition, quality leisure time spent with your family and friends is essential for mind, body, and spirit. It's vital to the building and maintenance of good relationships. When your children leave home, it's too late to regret the sports days you missed, the school plays you never went to, and the vacations you never had together. Unfortunately, the pressures of today's life are such that people find it increasingly difficult to set aside time for leisure.

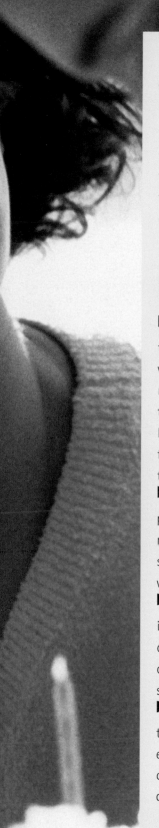

the enemies of leisure

The two great enemies of healthy leisure time are the television and the computer. Falling asleep in front of the evening movie the minute you've finished your meal or spending three hours after work on the Internet will not rebuild your health. It's not that long ago that the worst punishment for a child was being sent to their room but today, getting them out of their bedroom and away from the computer and games console is a major problem.

If you really want to give your health a boost, there are far better ways to spend your leisure time.

▶ Vacations. You may find that taking a long vacation can create almost more stress than remaining at work. A long vacation requires complex planning, and then you may worry constantly while you're away about the work still to be done and that you'll return to a bigger workload than ever. If this happens, it's often more beneficial to take 3- or 4-day breaks. But don't take your mobile phone and laptop with you, or leave a dozen contact numbers with the office. As you'd soon discover if you were fired, no-one is indispensable and if the business can't function without you for a while, then you and others are not doing the job properly.

▶ Learn a new skill. It may sound trite to say join the local theater group, go to painting classes, or learn a foreign language. But these are great ways of meeting new non-work-related people and of participating in activities that require a different set of skills. All this will help you take your mind off the trials and tribulations of your working life.

▶ Involve the family. If you have a family then some of your leisure activities must involve them too. It doesn't matter whether it's following a football team, going camping, doing jigsaw puzzles, or playing Scrabble together. Activities like these not only represent a huge investment in your physical health, but are an important supportive prop for the emotional health and well-being of your family unit.

▶ Make sure you're really having fun. Many people, even when they do make time in their busy schedules for leisure activities, are so afraid that they might be seen to be enjoying themselves that they fill this time with punishing exercise regimes, obsessional competitive games, or "team-building" activities. This is not leisure for pleasure and does nothing to improve your health. In fact, the reverse is true.

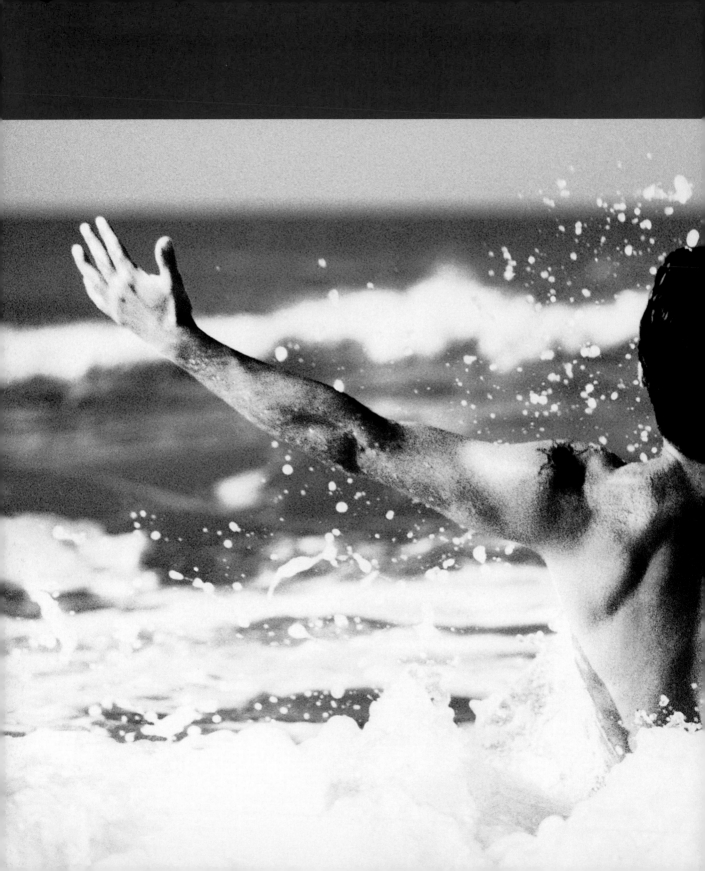

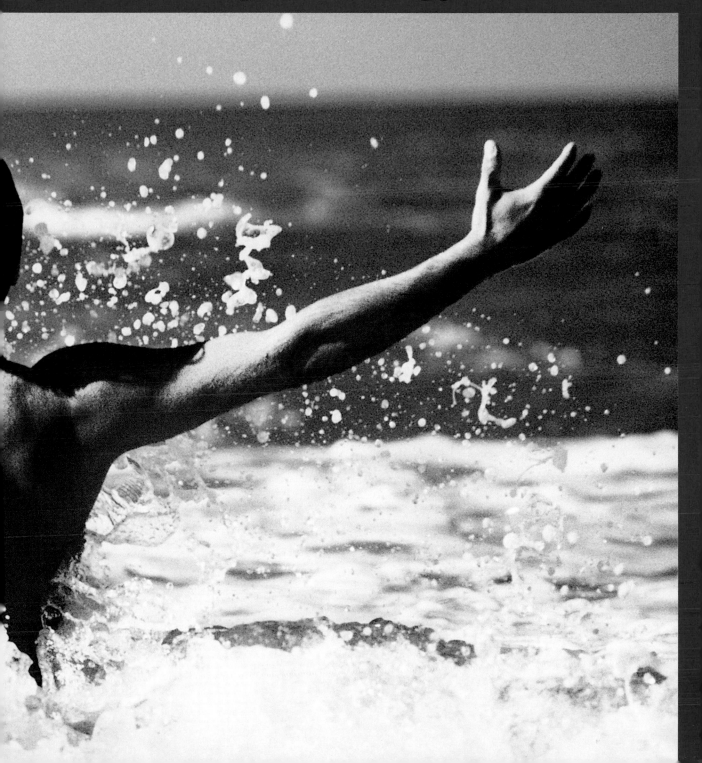

part 2 super energy detox

the search for super energy

Energy is the key to life, whether you think of it as a spiritual energy, a flowing life force like the chi of Chinese medicine, or the electrical impulses that scientists tell us govern every bodily function. Without an adequate supply of mental, spiritual, and physical energy, leading a full life becomes impossible and maintaining good health is out of the question.

Energy equates to vitality and we all know people whose boundless and unquenchable vitality seems to have no limits. These are the people who are the "doers," the creators, the rocks in an emergency, the steadfast friends in a crisis. But their performance is not built just on their goodwill, kindness, or humanity. Without the energy to follow through, their good intentions would fall at the first hurdle.

But millions of you wake up every morning feeling exhausted and worn out. In fact, tiredness is one of the most common problems that send you to your doctor. Overheated, stuffy buildings, and crowded public transportation take their toll. Who knows what else you catch when you catch your morning train? Traffic jams and bad weather turn even the most mild mannered into road-rage maniacs. And the depressing thought of another routine day in a frustrating job that you don't enjoy, the stresses of dealing with the public or a demanding, insensitive boss are enough to make you go straight back to bed and hide under the comforter.

Working moms often have a lot of extra pressures to cope with as well, and as if all this weren't enough on its own, when winter brings short days, lack of sunlight, and Seasonal Affective Disorder (SAD), the agony is just piled on.

In an ideal world we would all be living on a carefully balanced diet that keeps the baddies to a minimum and is chock-full of nutritious ingredients. My top twelve energy superfoods are baked potatoes, pasta, beans, rice, bananas, corn, fruit, oats, nuts and seeds, buckwheat, lentils, and, of course, bread. Whenever possible, eat these foods in their raw, "whole" and unprocessed state, and avoid adding fatty sauces, sugar, or too much butter. Nature has provided us with a powerhouse of energy-giving foods, so it makes sense to include plenty of them in a balanced diet. Sadly, we're so busy that few of us have the time or the energy to plan our shopping and eating in advance.

You need the Super Energy Detox. You'll be amazed at how quickly it will give you that surge of extra energy, an all-over glow of well-being, and a feeling of immense relief as the weight lifts from your shoulders and you return once again to being a fully functioning human being. Renewing your vital forces will help your body to overcome disease and damage, and your mind to deal with its problems. In fact, Super Energy Detox will help maintain both your physical and spiritual well-being in the state that is your birthright.

time to detox?

Zest, pizzazz, charisma, fit, "it," buzz, aura – all wonderful words that really mean energy. Are you blessed with it or do you constantly feel that your get up and go has got up and gone? Even if you think you've never had it, I can assure you that you can have it, and sooner than you think thanks to Super Energy Detox. To find out if you're an energy giant, and if not why not, answer these simple questions.

1 What do you do first thing in the morning?
- **A** I get up when I wake up.
- **B** I snooze for 10 minutes then get up.
- **C** I go back to sleep and wake up an hour later feeling dreadful.

2 How many hours sleep do you get a night?
- **A** 5 or 6.
- **B** less than 5.
- **C** more than 8.

3 Are you a snorer?
- **A** Not as far as I know.
- **B** Only if I have a cold or drink too much.
- **C** The neighbors bang on the wall most nights.

4 Do you take sleeping pills?
- **A** Never.
- **B** Rarely.
- **C** Every night.

5 How many cups of tea and coffee do you drink each day?
- **A** 4 or less without sugar.
- **B** 4–8 without sugar.
- **C** More than 8 without sugar (if you take sugar add 2 points per cup to your final score).

6 What is the total weight of sweets and chocolates you eat each day?
- **A** 4 ounces or less.
- **B** 4 to 8 ounces.
- **C** more than 8 ounces.

7 Do you (check as many as you like)
Smoke?
Drink more than 14 drinks (women) or 21 drinks (men) of alcohol a week?
Take tranquilizers or anti-depressants?
Use recreational drugs?

8 Which of the following sums up your exercise pattern?
- **A** No problems on that score. I'm at the gym most nights of the week.
- **B** I don't do much, but I probably get half an hour's exercise three or four times a week.
- **C** I don't do any if I can possibly avoid it.

9 How much time do you spend on your favorite hobby?
- **A** At least 4 hours a week.
- **B** Less than 4 hours a week.
- **C** I don't have time for hobbies.

10 When you come home from work, sit in the armchair, and watch your favorite show on TV, do you fall asleep in the middle?
- **A** Never.
- **B** Occasionally.
- **C** Nearly always.

11 Do you nod off at inappropriate moments, for example in the middle of dinner, at your office desk, during a work meeting, in the cinema or theater?
- **A** No.
- **B** Very rarely.
- **C** Embarrassingly often.

12 Do you feel exhausted most of the time?
- **A** No.
- **B** Only at the end of a long hard week.
- **C** All the time, even when I wake up in the morning.

13 Do you have chronic digestive problems like indigestion, irritable bowel syndrome, bloating, or gas?
- **A** Not at all.
- **B** Occasionally if I eat things that I know don't agree with me.
- **C** Yes, after almost every meal.

14 Do you eat regular meals on most days?
- **A** Usually, but it's not always possible.
- **B** Not very often as I'm too tired to bother when I get home.
- **C** Hardly ever. I don't have time for breakfast. I eat nibbles during the day and maybe have a takeout in the evening.

15 If somebody suggested you had a stressful life, what would you say?
- **A** Stressful? Never heard of the word.
- **B** Well, isn't everybody occasionally?
- **C** I haven't got time to answer that question – look at all the work I have to do.

Score:
> **A** – 1 point
> **B** – 3 points
> **C or check** – 5 points

Over 85 – your energy levels are at an all-time low and you're going to have to make a supreme effort just to get to the store to buy the ingredients for the energy detox that you need so urgently. You'll be amazed by the surge of energy you'll feel afterward. It'll give you the ability to make the serious changes to your lifestyle and diet – for instance, including regular amounts of all my recommended energy superfoods (see page 65) – that you need for a long-term solution to your lack of energy.

60–85 – you probably feel ok sometimes but when things pile up, your eating gets worse and you soon burn off your energy reserves and start to find life a struggle. Once you've tried energy detoxing, you'll see that you can even out these ups and downs and restore some balance to your life.

35–60 – you're the one who will have the energy and vitality to take on the challenge of detoxing right now, even though you need it least. Use the plans in this book and incorporate plenty of my recommended energy-rich foods, and everyone else will still have problems keeping up with you when you're in your eighties.

Under 35 – I'm glad I don't live with you. You're probably up at dawn and still clubbing at midnight. You've got boundless energy but I suspect there may be a bit too much. There is, after all, a difference between being super-energetic and hyperactive. Calm down a little and make some time to stand and stare.

cleansing for

If you're suffering from real exhaustion and chronic fatigue, you've just got to take the bull by the horns and follow my full three-day Cleansing for Energy detox followed by the eight-day return to normal eating.

For patients of mine who have struggled with a lack of energy for years, I advise that they aim to do this combination of programs four times a year. Once they've tried it they've found – as I'm sure you will too – that the benefits are so obvious and their energy has received such an enormous boost, that they're happy to stick to this pattern. And it's always a lot easier the second time around.

take care

While you're following the programs, it's really important to take my advice on the supplements you need (see page 70), and before you start, don't forget to check with your doctor to make sure the programs are suitable for you. If your lack of energy is not due to some serious underlying illness, there are few contra-indications.

energy

short of time?

If it's difficult to take a few days off – which you really need if you're going to do the full three-day program – then follow the twenty-four hour detox once a week or the forty-eight hour program once a month. You'll soon notice the benefits in an increase in your general energy and vitality.

And as a bonus, these Cleansing for Energy plans will boost your natural resistance to disease, significantly lower your blood pressure and cholesterol levels, improve your liver function, and help make you mentally more positive and alert.

side effects

You'll feel some side effects when you're fasting, even on a twenty-four hour program. The most common side effect is a headache; on forty-eight hour or three-day fasts you may also experience a "healing crisis." For detailed information on these side effects and how to manage them, see page 13.

the extras

My Cleansing for Energy plans are quite drastic and your body will need extra support to help it through. Even the eight-day return to normal eating regime is based on a fairly limited food intake, and although it does include a lot of high-nutrient foods, you'll need some extra support for this, too.

the supplements

There are three groups of supplements you need to take each day to help you on any of the programs.

supportive supplements to maintain nutrient levels

▶ A high potency multi-vitamin and mineral supplement (choose one of the reputable brand leaders)

▶ 500mg vitamin C, three times a day. If possible, take ester-C as it's non-acidic and less likely to cause digestive upsets, especially while you're on a restricted diet.

▶ A high-potency B-complex to nourish the central nervous system and stimulate energy conversion

supplements that help the body convert food into available energy

▶ Co-enzyme Q – a powerful anti-oxidant and especially valuable for chronic fatigue, glandular fever, tired-all-the-time syndrome, and M E

▶ Kelp – a major source of iodine. This controls the thyroid gland, which is vital for the production of energy.

supplements that directly increase the body's energy supply

▶ Guarana – the extraordinary herb used as a source of energy by the Indians of the Brazilian rainforest for more than a thousand years. It's unique in its ability to produce gradual slow-release, long-term energy, rather than the quick boost and let-down that you get from a cup of strong coffee or a can of cola.

▶ Ginseng – used by the Chinese as an energy medicine for more than six thousand years. It not only boosts physical and mental energy, but as a bonus helps increase natural immunity and the body's ability to resist the damaging effects of stress.

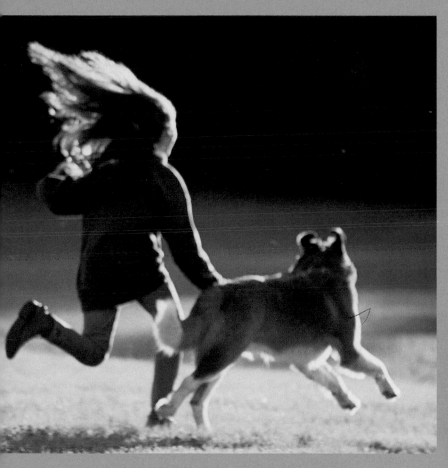

rest and relaxation

People are incredulous when I say that a combination of fasting and gentle exercise will help improve their energy levels – until they try it themselves. By giving your body a rest from high-fat, high-sugar foods, you'll find you can generate much more sustainable energy.

Detoxing does put some strain on your physical resources though, so it's essential to get enough rest while you're doing it. But there's a delicate balance to be struck. Sleeping late in the morning is fine, so is putting your feet up for 10 minutes a few times a day. But your body needs to be active. This will not only stimulate your heart, circulation, and breathing, and get your liver working, but it will trigger the release of the activity hormones that you're so obviously lacking.

And don't overdo the physical exertion in the belief that you'll be detoxing more effectively. You won't. Your body will just be producing toxic chemical by-products, which will defeat the whole object of detoxing. You'll also be draining your energy reserves. Two or three 15-minute walks a day are ideal. Jogging or going to the gym aren't.

what to drink

While you're detoxing you need to keep up your fluid intake. I always recommend drinking as much filtered water, low-mineral-content bottled water, or herb tea as you like, but not adding milk or sweetener. And canned drinks, fizzy water, black tea, coffee, and alcohol are definite no-nos, as are sugar-free commercial drinks since these contain artificial sweeteners.

twenty-four hour cleansing

The day before your twenty-four hour energy detox, avoid all animal protein and have a fairly light diet of just fruit, vegetables, and salads. Drink at least one and a half quarts of water and reduce your caffeine intake to lessen the likelihood of headaches on the following day. At bedtime take a natural bulk laxative like psyllium seeds or linseeds. You can certainly follow this twenty-four hour plan while you're at work, but it's easier if you have a day at home.

on waking   A large glass of hot water with a thick slice of organic unwaxed lemon

breakfast   A large glass of hot water with a thick slice of organic unwaxed lemon
A glass of unsweetened pineapple juice

mid-morning   A large glass of hot water with a thick slice of organic unwaxed lemon

lunch   A large glass of hot water with a thick slice of organic unwaxed lemon
A large glass of any unsalted vegetable juice
A mug of ginseng tea

mid-afternoon   A large glass of hot water with a thick slice of organic unwaxed lemon

supper   Mango, Kiwi, and Pineapple Juice (see recipe, page 191)
A mug of raspberry leaf tea

evening   A large glass of hot water with a thick slice of organic unwaxed lemon
Carrot, Apple, and Celery Juice (see recipe, page 187)

bedtime   A mug of camomile tea

forty-eight hour cleansing

Start by following the twenty-four hour Cleansing for Energy plan, then have:

on waking A large glass of hot water with a thick slice of organic unwaxed lemon

breakfast A large glass of hot water with a thick slice of organic unwaxed lemon and quarter of a
teaspoon of powdered cinnamon – this tends to float on top of the water even if you stir
A large bunch of grapes
A mug of lemon and ginger tea

mid-morning A large glass of hot water with a thick slice of organic unwaxed lemon

lunch An apple, a stalk of celery, and 6 radishes
A large glass of tomato juice
A mug of mint tea

mid-afternoon A large glass of hot water with a thick slice of organic unwaxed lemon

supper A mango, $\frac{1}{2}$ cup blueberries, and a pear
4 prunes
A glass of unsalted mixed vegetable juice

evening A large glass of hot water with a thick slice of organic unwaxed lemon
Hauser Broth (see recipe, page 233)

bedtime A mug of camomile tea with a teaspoon of organic honey

three-day cleansing

When it comes to boosting your energy levels, it really does pay to go straight into the three-day Cleansing for Energy detox plan if at all possible. When you wake up on the morning of day 4, you'll feel like a new person – full of vim and vigor and raring to get on with life. Be careful though. The temptation to do all those things you've been putting off for months must be resisted, otherwise you'll dissipate all the benefits for which you've worked so hard. Take things gently and ease yourself gradually back into your normal routine.

The three-day cleansing is serious detoxing and you really can't do it and continue with your usual work. You'll also need at least one rest day afterwards to allow your system to return to normal, so this is where a day on the sofa will come in handy.

As a naturopath, I've used this plan for my patients for almost 40 years and although it's not strictly speaking a complete fast, it's the nearest you can safely get to one without professional supervision. These three days are very low in calories but you will be surprised at how soon you stop feeling hungry. To help overcome the hunger pangs, take two teaspoons of the Swiss herbal tonic BioStrath Elixir, three times a day, and don't forget your supportive and energy-boosting supplements (see page 70).

On days 1 and 2, follow the forty-eight hour Cleansing for Energy plan. Day 3 is an animal-protein- and dairy-product-free day that will optimize the energy-giving benefits of the first two days.

Days 1 and 2, follow the Forty-Eight Hour Cleansing program. Day 3:

on waking   A large glass of hot water with a thick slice of organic unwaxed lemon

breakfast   A large glass of hot water with a thick slice of organic unwaxed lemon
Half a cantaloupe filled with fresh berries
A mug of rosehip tea

mid-morning   Carrot, Apple, and Beet Juice (see recipe, page 188)

lunch   A large glass of hot water with a thick slice of organic unwaxed lemon
A bowl of Porridge with Cinnamon and Dried Fruits made with water (see recipe, page 182)
A large glass of tomato juice

mid-afternoon   A large glass of hot water with a thick slice of organic unwaxed lemon

supper   A large glass of hot water with a thick slice of organic unwaxed lemon
A mixture of chopped steamed leek, cabbage, spinach, and kale, drizzled with olive oil
and lemon juice and with a generous sprinkling of nutmeg
A large glass of carrot juice
A mug of mint tea

evening   4 each dried or soaked prunes and apricots

bedtime   1 slice of whole-wheat bread with a little honey
A mug of mint tea

eight-day return to normal eating

You really must try to follow this eight-day plan immediately after the three-day detox. Doing so will maximize your energy gain and help your digestive system return to normal in a measured and gradual way. If you're not able to follow the plan exactly, then for at least three days after the three-day detox, try to avoid all animal protein and dairy products, and stick to a diet of raw or cooked fruit, vegetables, and salads, together with modest amounts of bread, potatoes, rice, and pasta. You should then introduce small amounts of the other food groups gradually over the next two or three days.

While you're following the eight-day plan, you may swap whole days around, or eat your main meal at lunchtime and your light meal in the evening, if that suits you, but don't take one meal from one day and one from another as you could end up with an imbalance in your diet. It's also a good idea to take a teaspoon of the Swiss herbal tonic BioStrath Elixir three times a day for a bit of extra support.

drinking habits

Having gotten into the habit of drinking much more fluid than you were probably used to before, try to continue, as fluid improves the efficiency of your digestive system and the amount of essential nutrients that your body absorbs from your food. And as before, you should keep on drinking a minimum of one and a half quarts a day of still mineral water, filtered tap water, or herb teas. And now that you've gotten used to starting your day with hot water and lemon, you should try to continue.

day 1
breakfast An orange, half a grapefruit, a large slice of melon
A glass of unsalted vegetable juice
A mug of herb tea

light meal   A plateful of raw red and yellow bell peppers, cucumber, tomato, broccoli, cauliflower, celery, carrots, radishes, and lots of fresh parsley, dressed with extra-virgin olive oil and lemon juice
A large glass of unsweetened fruit juice

main meal   A large mixed salad of lettuce, tomato, watercress, onion, garlic, beets, celeriac, fresh mint, and any herbs you like, with extra-virgin olive oil and lemon juice
A large glass of unsweetened fruit juice or unsalted vegetable juice

day 2

breakfast   A bowl of Porridge with Cinnamon and Dried Fruits made with water (see recipe, page 182)
A large glass of Mango, Kiwi, and Pineapple Juice (see recipe, page 191)

light meal   Half an avocado, sliced, with watercress, tomatoes, and cucumber, on mixed leaves with a generous squeeze of lemon juice
A whole-wheat roll
2 kiwi fruit
A large glass of unsalted vegetable juice

main meal   A large bowl of Vegetable, Bean, and Barley Soup (see recipe, page 232)
A large slice of melon and a bunch of grapes

day 3

breakfast   Real Swiss Muesli (see recipe, page 182)
A glass of half-orange, half-grapefruit juice

light meal   Papaya and Watercress Salad (see recipe, page 242)
1 slice of whole-wheat bread and 2 tablespoons of Hummus (see recipe, page 242)
An apple

main meal   Spanish Omelette (see recipe, page 206) with a mixed green salad
Spiced Baked Apple (see recipe, page 246)
A large glass of hot water with a thick slice of organic unwaxed lemon

day 4

It's vital for your system that you follow this "rice" day exactly as it's laid out since it's an important part of your cleansing and energizing treatment. The most convenient way of going about it is to prepare the rice you need for the whole day, so start by cooking $^3/_4$ cup brown rice in 2 cups of water, or half in water and the remaining half in vegetable stock for a more savory flavor. In addition, make sure you drink at least an extra four large glasses of water during the day.

breakfast $^1/_2$ cup cooked rice with $^2/_3$ cup stewed apple flavored with honey, cinnamon, and grated lemon rind
A large glass of hot water with a thick slice of organic unwaxed lemon

mid-morning   A large glass of hot water with a thick slice of organic unwaxed lemon

lunch $^1/_2$ cup cooked rice with $1^1/_2$ cups steamed vegetables – celery, leek, carrot, tomato, spinach, broccoli and shredded cabbage

mid-afternoon   A large glass of hot water with a thick slice of organic unwaxed lemon

supper $^1/_2$ cup cooked rice mixed with soaked dried apricots and raisins, and the flesh of a pink grapefruit
A large glass of hot water with a thick slice of organic unwaxed lemon

bedtime   A mug of camomile tea with a teaspoon of organic honey

day 5

breakfast   Half a pink grapefruit, baked beans (make sure you buy organic low-salt, low-sugar beans) on whole-wheat toast with a large poached or grilled tomato

light meal   Italian Toast (see recipe, page 206)
Dried Fruit Compôte – make enough for 2 meals (see recipe, page 246)

main meal   Green Pasta with Tuna Fish (see recipe, page 205)
Half a pineapple with 2 tablespoons of sour cream and any fresh berries

day 6

breakfast Dried Fruit Compôte (see recipe, page 246) with low-fat live yogurt and an orange

light meal Gratin of Potatoes – no they're not fattening! – and Mushrooms
(see recipe, page 207)
A glass of Carrot, Apple, and Beet Juice (see recipe, page 188)

main meal Cabbage Soup with Potatoes (see recipe, page 232)
Tuna and Mixed Bean Salad (see recipe, page 241)
An apple and a pear

day 7

breakfast 2 hot whole-wheat rolls with a little butter
A banana and a large glass of orange juice

light meal A large portion of Red, White, and Green Coleslaw (see recipe, page 240) with cottage
cheese
A peach or nectarine or 3 fresh apricots

main meal Non-Meatballs in Tomato Sauce (see recipe, page 213) with pasta and Tomato and Red
Onion Salad (see recipe, page 241)
Mango and Kiwi Sorbet (see recipe, page 248)

day 8

breakfast Scrambled Eggs with Smoked Salmon (see recipe, page 183)
1 thin slice of whole-wheat toast
Juice of a lemon in a large glass of water

light meal Papaya and Watercress Salad (see recipe, page 242)
2 rye crispbreads with a matchbox-size piece of Brie

main meal Cold Beet and Apple Soup (see recipe, page 232)
Spiced Chickpea Casserole (see recipe, page 208)
A fresh fruit salad

replenishing for

All your efforts in completing the cleansing detox will be wasted if you just return to your old bad habits, so what you need now is to make up your energy deficit and replenish your depleted stores. It's extremely important that you resist the temptation to take the easy way out and stuff yourself on high-energy foods and drinks. All these do is provide large amounts of sugar and little else.

From now on, you need to plan your eating so that your energy supplies always match your energy requirements as closely as possible. That's the way to avoid getting back into your old habits. You only need to run out of gas at three o'clock in the morning once in your life to make sure that you keep your tank filled for ever after. And I hope you've now learned the same lesson regarding your body's fuel tank.

the importance of mental energy

Most people fail to recognize that mental energy and physical energy are equally important. While your physical energy can be replenished through the sugar in your bloodstream, you can also replenish your reserves of mental energy.

The first step is to learn to be more assertive and to actually say "no" when people ask you to take on extra jobs at home or work. So on weekends, don't commit yourself to endless fix-it projects, helping your best friend to move, or cutting your mother- in-law's grass. If you've got a yard, sit in it with a long drink and a good book. Go for a picnic or a walk in the countryside, or see a film or a concert. In other words, get yourself some spiritual as well as physical sustenance.

energy

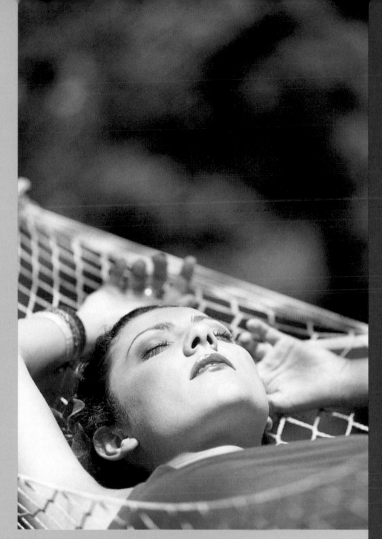

Most of us find it hard to say "no," but you have to learn to do so. When you do, it may come as a shock to your friends, colleagues, and family as they're probably used to you being the one who's always there to help out. But try it and you'll be thrilled at how quickly your initial guilt turns to relief and then to self-congratulation.

And as well as making fewer commitments and so less pressure, what you also need now to help you replenish your energy is plenty of good quality sleep. Once or twice a week have an early supper, a long soak in the bath, and be in bed by nine o'clock. Even if you read or listen to the radio in bed, the extra hours of relaxation that you'll enjoy will deliver an energy-boosting charge to your system.

energy through relaxation

Relaxation exercises and meditation are other great ways to replenish your energy. I give some suggested exercises on pages 110–113, but it's worth looking at these now and getting in a little practice as these techniques get much easier with regular use and will help you at this stage of your energizing process as well as later on.

seven-day replenishing

The foods of the next seven days will supply you with both instant- and slow-release energy. This means that your metabolic processes will generate the power necessary for the essential bodily functions, for your immediate physical needs and to build up the surplus that's necessary for your reserve supplies. It's these reserves that help your body cope with sudden emergencies, the unexpected extra demands that crop up every day.

It's important during this week that you eat a little less at a time and do it more often. And to guarantee as wide a spread as possible of energy-giving nutrients, you have to avoid eating the same foods every day. As with the eight-day return to normal eating, if it suits your lifestyle, you can swap a day's meals around, or you can swap whole days, but don't mix meals from different days.

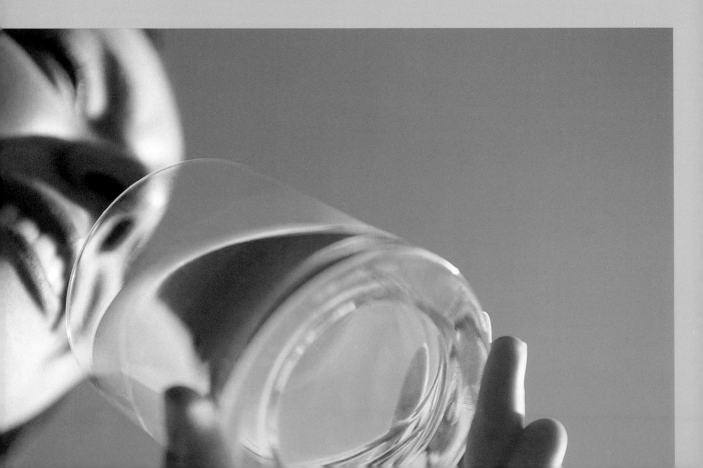

time for a drink

Continue to drink at least one and a half quarts a day, of which at least one quart must be water, and you can also now drink a total of five cups of real tea and coffee, but not more than three of coffee. Some alcohol's allowed, but don't exceed 14 drinks a week (women) or 21 (men), and carry on avoiding energy-robbing high-sugar canned fizzy drinks.

added extras

Carry on taking your guarana, co-enzyme Q, ginseng and vitamin B complex supplements, but now add the following three:

▶ Chromium picolinate helps balance insulin levels
▶ Kelp contains iodine, which you need if your thyroid gland is under-performing
▶ BioStrath Elixir, the universally available Swiss natural herbal tonic.

day 1

breakfast   Real Swiss Muesli (see recipe, page 182) and 1 slice of whole-wheat toast with honey

mid-morning   A selection of dried fruits and fresh unsalted nuts

light meal   Whole-wheat bread, a selection of cheeses, radishes, celery, and fresh fruit

mid-afternoon   A banana

main meal   Large Grilled Shrimp on Salad Leaves (see recipe, page 204) with a salad of avocado, spinach, and toasted pumpkin seeds
Fresh fruit

day 2

breakfast   Dried Fruit Compôte (see recipe, page 246)

mid-morning   A matchbox-size piece of cheese and an apple

light meal   Hummus and Guacamole (see recipes, page 242) with hot whole-wheat pita and a selection of crudités

mid-afternoon   A mixture of raisins and unsalted, unroasted peanuts

main meal   Spicy Energy Beans (see recipe, page 209)
Tomato and Red Onion Salad (see recipe, page 241)

day 3
breakfast   Carrot, Apple, and Celery Juice (see recipe, page 187), 2 boiled eggs and 2 slices of whole-wheat toast with butter

mid-morning   Yogurt and Strawberry Smoothie (see recipe, page 187)

light meal   Leek and Potato Soup (see recipe, page 233) with whole-wheat bread and a bunch of grapes

mid-afternoon   Pita bread and Hummus (see recipe, page 242)

main meal   Steak in Red Wine (see recipe, page 209)

day 4
breakfast   Buckwheat Crêpes (see recipe, page 184)

mid-morning   Rye crispbread with cottage cheese and a few dates

light meal   Mediterranean Omelette Flan (see recipe, page 204)

mid-afternoon   Greek yogurt with a teaspoon of honey and sunflower seeds

main meal   Millet and Mushroom Risotto (see recipe, page 207)
Spiced Baked Apple (see recipe, page 246)

day 5
breakfast   Scrambled Eggs with Smoked Salmon (see recipe, page 183) on whole-wheat toast
A glass of half-orange and half-grapefruit juice

mid-morning	Dried fruit with fresh unsalted nuts
light meal	Gratin of Potatoes and Mushrooms (see recipe, page 207)
mid-afternoon	Energy Teabread (see recipe, page 182)
main meal	Dutch Chicken (see recipe, page 205) with rice Honeyed Plums (see recipe, page 247) with mascarpone cheese

day 6

breakfast	A glass of tomato juice, fresh fruit salad, a carton of live yogurt and 1 slice of whole-wheat toast
mid-morning	Apple, Peanut, and Banana Smoothie (see recipe, page 187)
light meal	Tuna and Mixed Bean Salad (see recipe, page 241)
mid-afternoon	Dried Fruit Compôte (see recipe, page 246)
main meal	Baked Cod with Sesame Seeds (see recipe, page 201) Mango and Kiwi Sorbet (see recipe, page 248)

day 7

breakfast	Savory Toastie (see recipe, page 184)
mid-morning	Energy Teabread (see recipe, page 182)
light meal	Chillied Sardine Sandwich (see recipe, page 209) with cherry tomatoes and watercress
mid-afternoon	A small bowl of Real Swiss Muesli (see recipe, page 182)
main meal	Beef and Ginger Stir-Fry (see recipe, page 223) served on a bed of noodles Banana and Mango Crumble (see recipe, page 247)

rebuilding for

At last, the moment you've been waiting for – when you start to rebuild your energy and generate a pattern that will sustain you in the future. These next steps will lay the foundations for achieving Super Energy for Life.

the bad guys/good guys swap box

One thing you can do to help you improve your energy levels is to make some simple changes to your normal eating habits. When it comes to food, there are good guys and bad guys. Choosing to eat the good guys will start you on the road to rebuilding your energy faster than you think, but there is an important added bonus. By reducing the amount of high-fat, high-salt, high-sugar foods that you consume on a regular basis and by increasing your consumption of whole grains, nuts, seeds, and complex carbohydrates, you reduce your risk of heart disease, circulatory disorders, and many types of cancer.

BAD GUYS	GOOD GUYS
Sugar-coated cereals	Oatmeal, granola, whole-grain cereal
Eggrolls, chimichangas, salamis	Fish, organic beef, lamb, poultry
Cookies, sweets, chocolates	Dried fruit, bananas
French fries	Baked or boiled potatoes
Salty snacks	Fresh nuts and seeds
Sliced white bread	Organic whole-grain or rye
Convenience foods	Simple home cooking
Burgers and hot dogs	Veggie pizza, shish kebab in pita
Squashes, fizzy drinks	Water, fresh juices

There's more detail on a simple but effective strate for changing your diet long term on page 47.

energy

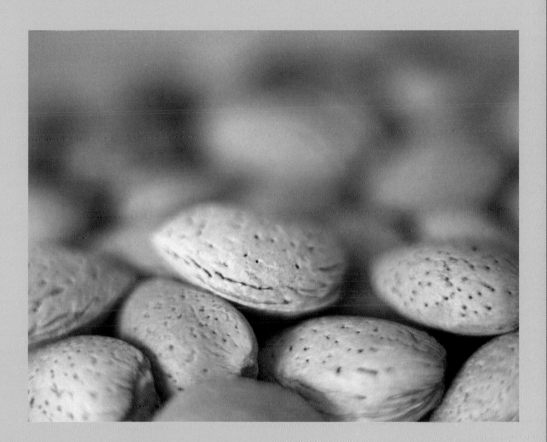

the zinc problem

Chronic fatigue has become an epidemic. If you've suffered exhaustion for several weeks, you must see your doctor in case an underlying medical condition like anemia, a thyroid problem, or diabetes is responsible. Zinc deficiency is a common cause of exhaustion (and skin problems, see page 138), but excessive tiredness is also a symptom of depression, so many doctors are likely to prescribe anti-depressants. But anti-depressants interfere with the body's absorption of zinc, so you end up in a vicious circle. Forewarned is forearmed.

fourteen-day rebuilding

Start this Rebuilding for Energy regime with the seven-day Replenishing for Energy eating plan. It will help get you into the right frame of mind as well as into the routine of eating properly for energy. In other words, it will introduce you to the concept of grazing, which helps you maintain a constant blood-sugar level and so avoid the ups and downs that drain your energy resources so severely.

Throughout this second week you may choose any of the mid-morning or mid-afternoon snacks from the first week – but please don't just rely on your favorite two or three. Ringing the changes spreads your nutritional input so you obtain the optimum amounts of essential vitamins, minerals, and protective plant chemicals. As before, you can swap a day's meals around, or you can swap whole days, but don't mix meals from different days. Continue taking your Replenishing for Energy supplements throughout this program.

drinks

▶ As with the Replenishing for Energy program, still maintain a high level of fluid intake – at least one and a half quarts a day, one quart of which should be water.

▶ Black tea and real coffee are allowed, but not more than five cups a day and certainly not more than three cups of coffee – avoiding instant decaffeinated coffee of course.

▶ Some alcohol is still allowed, but not more than 14 drinks a week for a woman, 21 for a man.

▶ Don't drink canned fizzy drinks of any kind. They're either full of energy-robbing sugar or full of chemical artificial sweeteners. Yuck!

Days 1–7, follow the Seven-Day Replenishing program.

day 8

breakfast   Porridge with Cinnamon and Dried Fruits (see recipe, page 182)
1 slice of whole-wheat toast with a scraping of butter
A banana
A glass of orange juice

light meal   Avocado, Tomato, and Mozzarella Salad (see recipe, page 243)

main meal   Traditional Chicken Soup (see recipe, page 228)
Squash, Almond, and Raisin Bulgur (see recipe, page 225)
Dried Fruit Compôte (see recipe, page 246)

day 9

breakfast   Lightly cooked fresh fruit compôte of strawberries, raspberries, currants, blackberries,
blueberries, and apple with plain live yogurt
A boiled egg
1 slice of whole-wheat toast with butter

light meal   Channel Island Potato Salad (see recipe, page 243)
A piece of fresh fruit

main meal   Posh Cauliflower Cheese with Pasta (see recipe, page 208)
Tomato and Red Onion Salad (see recipe, page 241)
Orange and Mango Fool (see recipe, page 247)

day 10

breakfast   A whole pink grapefruit
3–4 canned sardines (in olive oil) mashed with black pepper and lemon juice, spread on 2
slices of whole-wheat toast and covered with sliced tomato

light meal   Pasta all'Aglio e Olio (see recipe, page 197) with a mixed green salad

main meal   1 slice of fresh honeydew or cantaloupe melon
Roman Liver (see recipe, page 211) with snap beans and carrots
Multi-grain crackers, goat's cheese, and a bunch of grapes

day 11
breakfast   A glass of half-orange, half-grapefruit juice
Real Swiss Muesli (see recipe, page 182) sprinkled with a teaspoon each of sunflower,
sesame, and pumpkin seeds

light meal   Whole-wheat pita stuffed with tomato, cucumber, radishes, green onion, shredded lettuce,
celery, watercress, and olives, with a drizzle of good extra-virgin olive oil and a
sprinkling of oregano
A piece of fresh fruit

main meal   A glass of tomato juice
Baked Cod with Sesame Seeds (see recipe, page 201) on a bed of spinach
Bread and Tomato Salad (see recipe, page 240)
A bowl of fresh strawberries

day 12
breakfast   A glass of beet juice
Mushrooms on Whole-wheat Toast (see recipe, page 183)

light meal   A large baked potato filled with baked beans
A glass of pineapple juice
Fresh cherries and a bunch of grapes

main meal   Grilled Lamb Chops with Rosemary (see recipe, page 210) with boiled new potatoes in
their skins and kale
Dried Fruit Compôte (see recipe, page 246) with Greek yogurt

day 13

breakfast   Fresh orange, pink grapefruit, tangerine, and kiwi slices with natural live yogurt, sprinkled with a tablespoon of sliced almonds and a drizzle of honey
Poached Kipper and Tomato (see recipe, page 185)
1 slice of whole-wheat toast

light meal   Lamb and Pine Nut Koftas (see recipe, page 223) with a salad of watercress, mint, and chopped onion

main meal   Brown Rice Risotto with Sun-dried Tomatoes (see recipe, page 210) served with Spanish Salad (see recipe, page 241)
Spiced Baked Apple (see recipe, page 246)

day 14

breakfast   English Breakfast the Healthy Way (see recipe, page 185)

light meal   Ten-Minute Mussels (see recipe, page 225) with crusty French bread
A pear

main meal   Duck Breasts with Pepper Sauce (see recipe, page 211) served with Grilled Italian Vegetables (see recipe, page 211)
A peach

energy lifeplan

It's inevitable that you will experience an occasional attack of the energy-droops – late nights, a few drinks too many, extra pressure at work, problems at home, or even the after-effects of a cold or of an attack of flu. If you're healthy you'll soon recover from these episodes, or you could give yourself a detox to get back on your feet sooner.

But to avoid regular and frequent dips, you need to plan your life for energy. It doesn't matter whether it's the energy you need for your day-to-day activities at home, for that immediate burst of extra zap required for a particularly hard day at work, or enough energy to extract maximum pleasure and enjoyment from your leisure activities.

Whatever your requirements, this section will tell you how to keep your body's supplies of essential vitality at a constant level. No more peaks and valleys. No more periods of being mentally hyper – the only way you've been able to cope in the past but it drives everyone around you crazy. No more superhuman efforts to drag yourself up from the depths of total exhaustion and conceal your chronic fatigue by putting on a brave face.

The lifestyle changes for energy at home, work, and leisure that I suggest will help you generate all the energy you need and will ensure that you've always got a bit in reserve for emergencies.

ten-point plan for lifestyle changes at home for energy

To achieve your goal of a high-energy home life you may need to follow all ten of these steps or you may need just a few of them. They're simple and effective and won't make too many demands on your already low energy levels.

1 Clear the clutter – there is nothing so fatiguing as living in a constant muddle. Fight against the packrat instinct and stop being a hoarder. Get rid of stuff you don't need.

2 Make sure your home is well ventilated and turn the heating down a couple of degrees. More fresh air and a cooler temperature help generate more physical energy.

3 Think about redecorating. Drab colors make for drab people – beige is enervating. You don't have to use crimson and gold, but lively colors generate their own energy.

4 Check all heating appliances annually, as low levels of carbon monoxide from unserviced heaters are a common cause of chronic fatigue and high levels could be fatal.

5 Fresh flowers in the house are great givers of energy – a vase of daffodils in the spring, wild flowers in the summer, a few twigs of autumn leaves, or a bowl of scented hyacinths at Christmas are all signs of nature's vigor.

6 Turn your bathroom into a spa by adding invigorating essential oils like rosemary, pine, or eucalyptus to your bath.

7 Cold baths or showers are very stimulating and push the body into producing extra energy. When you've finished washing, slowly add cold water to the bath while rubbing your arms, legs, and stomach briskly with a rough washcloth or loofah. If you're having a shower, turn the temperature down gradually. Once the water is really cold, stay in it for at least 10 seconds then dry yourself as briskly as possible with a rough towel. You may think it sounds awful, but once you've tried it you'll be hooked.

8 Scent your home with genuine herbal potpourri and banish forever artificially scented air fresheners, fake aromatherapy candles, and room deodorizers – the synthetic musk perfumes they contain are all toxic and de-energizing.

9 A good night's sleep is vital for energy at home, so make sure your bedroom has curtains that exclude all light and if necessary put lightproof roller blinds behind them.

10 Check your mattress. In 20 years you may have bought five toasters, three irons, and six cars, and still be sleeping on the same mattress. Once it sags, it won't support you properly and you won't get the restful, energy-generating sleep you need.

the power of breakfast

While you sleep your body is working hard as this is the time for growth and repair. Your brain switches off the activity hormones and turns on to maintenance mode. While all this work is going on you are using up your reserves of vital nutrients, so your storehouse needs replenishing, which is why breakfast is the most important meal of the day.

The ancient proverb "Breakfast like a king, lunch like a prince, dine like a pauper" has more than a grain of truth in it, but sadly most people today skip breakfast altogether. This is really bad news as ideally you should be getting 25 percent of your day's calories from breakfast. It is exactly what it says, breaking your fast, and for most people the time they spend in bed is the longest period they go without food. When you get up in the morning it may be 8–12 hours since you last ate and your blood-sugar level is at rock bottom. In order for your brain to function properly it needs a constant supply of sugar, which is why starting your day with breakfast is so important.

Skipping breakfast means poorer performance by schoolchildren, a greater risk of accidents when driving, and a lack of efficiency at work. It also means irritability.

scary statistics

Five million people in the United Kingdom alone don't bother to eat breakfast but grab a snack while dashing to work. Then they consume one and a half million bacon sandwiches, over a million bags of potato chips, more than a million sugary soft drinks, and half a million bags of sweets or bars of chocolate. Worse still, half of people at work don't eat anything for breakfast at all.

breakfast rules

What you eat for breakfast depends on your needs for that particular morning. Replenishing your protein means real energy and brain activity, whereas a mainly starch-based breakfast keeps you calm, serene, and happy.

the sporting breakfast

If you exercise early in the day, the essential ingredient in your breakfast should be lots of healthy calories and a fairly modest amount of protein, so the ideal start for you is a large bowl of hot cereal or granola with three prunes, three dried apricots, a handful of raisins and a generous sprinkling of mixed sunflower and pumpkin seeds for extra minerals. Follow with a matchbox-size piece of cheese and an apple, and take a banana with you to replace the energy and potassium after your exercise.

the expectant breakfast

Pregnancy isn't the time to think about dieting. As well as extra energy you need extra nutrients. A small pot of plain live yogurt with 2 teaspoons of honey drizzled on the top, and a sprinkling of mixed chopped, unsalted, unroasted fresh nuts will get you off to a good start in the morning. This will provide energy, protein, calcium, vitamin E, and lots of other essential nutrients. Follow with at least one thick slice of good whole-wheat or rye toast spread with organic peanut butter – yes, it's extremely healthy and a great source of instant energy – and a glass of fresh unsweetened fruit juice or unsalted vegetable juice.

the business power breakfast

If you're straight into a high-powered meeting that requires your brain to be bursting with energy, you need a high-protein breakfast, but avoid the traditional high-fat, high-cholesterol, artery-clogging frying pan breakfast, and skip the waffles and cream. Poached eggs, griddled bacon, a broiled low-fat sausage with grilled tomatoes and mushrooms, a glass of juice, and two slices of good whole-wheat toast will get you off to a flying start. The protein will stimulate your brain activity and energetic thought and you'll be unstoppable!

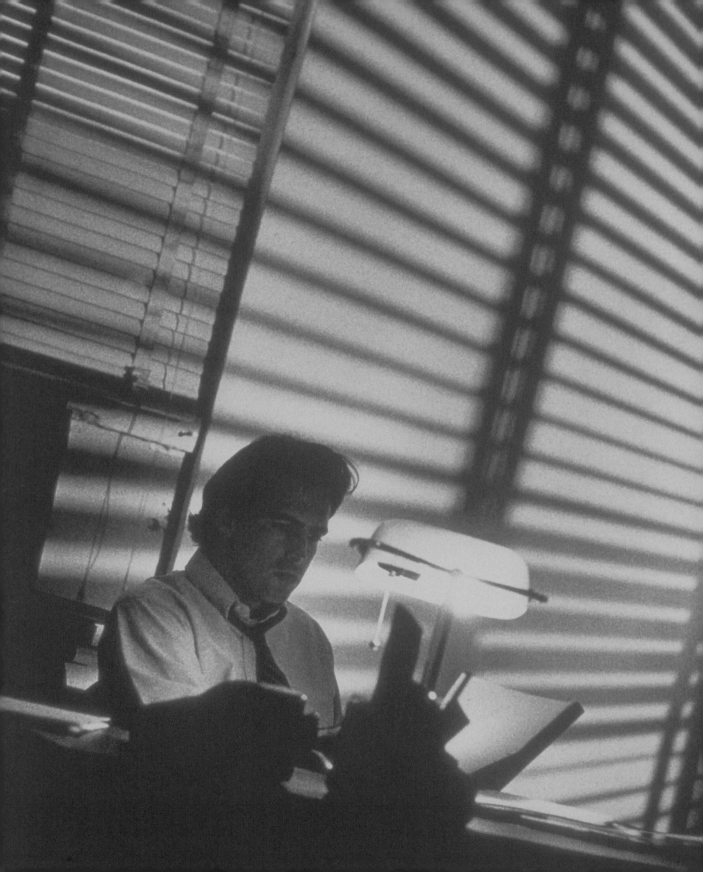

lifestyle changes at work

Everyone needs energy to do their job and depending on what you do, it may be physical energy, mental energy or, in most situations, a combination of the two. It's impossible to perform at your optimum level if you're constantly tired, but this is all too common a situation for many people in the workplace.

Assuming there's no underlying medical cause for your lack of energy, it's nearly always the result of a poor working environment, bad working posture, ergonomically wrong workstations and equipment or, all too commonly, just plain boredom. If you dislike your job, it's hard to summon up any enthusiasm. If you have to put up with bullying or sexual harassment from colleagues or superiors, you will inevitably be depressed, and fatigue goes hand in hand with depression.

Nutrition plays a vital role in the production of usable energy, and at work nutrition is even more important. You must not let the pressures of the job prevent you eating at regular intervals and you won't manage to break through the fatigue barrier if you're constantly relying on high-sugar snacks to give you an artificial energy boost (see pages 116–119).

Everyone wants to enjoy the satisfaction of a job well done and to achieve it you need to work in the most efficient way. To do that you must have energy in abundance and this will only be generated when you're reasonably happy and able to work in comfort.

ten-point plan for lifestyle changes at work for energy

Here's your ten-point plan for lifestyle changes that will maximize your energy at work.

1 All high-energy work days must start with a good breakfast.

2 With air conditioning in the summer and central heating in the winter, most work places are drier than the Sahara desert. This causes you to dehydrate and nothing saps your energy as quickly. Make sure you drink at least one and a half quarts of water between arriving at work and going home. You'll feel more comfortable generally and will be less at risk of headaches, which are exhausting in themselves.

3 Electronic machinery such as computers and printers pump out ozone and tiny particulates of carbon which irritate the eyes, lungs, and other mucus membranes. Create your own micro-climate by surrounding your workspace with loads of green plants, particularly ivies and spider plants. Plants not only give off moisture, which increases humidity and makes the atmosphere more comfortable, but they absorb pollutants too.

4 Always switch off electrical appliances when they're not being used. If you leave them in standby mode, they still produce ozone. The increase in your energy levels will more than compensate for the moments you have to wait for them to warm up.

5 If you use a computer for long periods you need a kitchen timer. Set it for 30 minutes and when it pings, sit back in your chair, look out of the window or across the room, and give your eyes and brain a 2-minute break. In addition, make sure you look away from the screen for at least 30 seconds every 15 minutes and focus your eyes on a distant object.

6 If your job frequently requires you to use a keyboard and the telephone at the same time, you must insist on having a hands-free headset. Keeping the telephone wedged between your ear and your shoulder while you access or input data is an almost certain guarantee of headaches, stiff necks, painful shoulders, backache, and constant fatigue.

7 You must take the time to organize your desk or workstation to suit you – it's no good having the telephone on the right-hand side if you're left-handed. Make sure you have an ergonomic chair that is fully adjustable to suit your size and shape, and that you have a footstool. This will maximize your comfort, minimize muscular effort, and conserve your much-needed energy.

8 Take the opportunity of your lunch break to recharge your energy reserves. Don't sit at your desk with a sandwich but get out of the office, even if it is raining. A short walk stimulates your circulation and breathing, which increases oxygen levels and stimulates your metabolism to produce more energy.

9 As well as eating all the energy superfoods (see pages 64–65), you must also eat to beat office pollution. That's not just chemicals and irritants, but also the myriad viruses and bacteria that circulate through the heating and cooling systems. To boost your natural resistance and protect you against infections that will drastically reduce your energy levels, eat a generous portion of at least two of these foods every day: carrots, red or yellow bell peppers, apricots, strawberries, blackberries, blueberries, spinach, watercress, spring greens, broccoli, sweet potatoes, cantaloupe, tomatoes, and dark green or red lettuce.

10 When you sit for long periods, your entire circulatory system slows down. This reduces the supply of oxygen to the brain and is a major contributor to office fatigue. Get into the habit of standing up during telephone calls. Shift your weight from foot to foot, do some gentle knee bends, take a few steps each way, stand on tiptoe a few times – all of this works the muscle pump in your calves and stimulates better blood flow.

last but not least

It's all too easy to forget that mental energy is as important as physical energy at work. Just as a 10-minute catnap can restore your physical activity levels, so a few minutes spent in simple meditation can stimulate an immediate increase in your mental energy. Surprisingly, this type of mental and spiritual relaxation doesn't leave you feeling down and sleepy, but can help set you up for the rest of the day's work (see pages 112–113).

lifestyle changes at leisure

We often equate leisure with relaxation and unwinding, which is quite proper, as it should be both. But it is important to understand that by using your leisure time constructively, you can really recharge your body's batteries. This process not only generates the immediate energy you need to enjoy your leisure pursuits, but also fills your energy tank to overflowing, allowing the surplus to be carried over into your home and working life.

I have discussed in detail the vital relationship between leisure, pleasure, and health on pages 60–61. But without a shadow of doubt, if you want to stimulate and release both your mental and physical energy, the key is how you spend your leisure time.

Ideally you should cultivate a combination of intellectual and physical leisure activities. This gives you a holistic energy boost that activates mind and body. After all, it's not much use if the spirit is willing but the flesh is weak, or conversely, if you're bursting with physical energy and so mentally exhausted that you can't even take the first step.

Chairman Mao was fond of saying that a march of a thousand miles begins with a single step. Bear this in mind and use it as the spur you need to take that first step into a new world of energy-boosting leisure activities. Don't worry about how you'll cope after 5 miles. Just focus on putting one foot in front of the other. You'll be surprised at how quickly you become absorbed in what you're doing, and that will be the beginning of the regeneration of your energy.

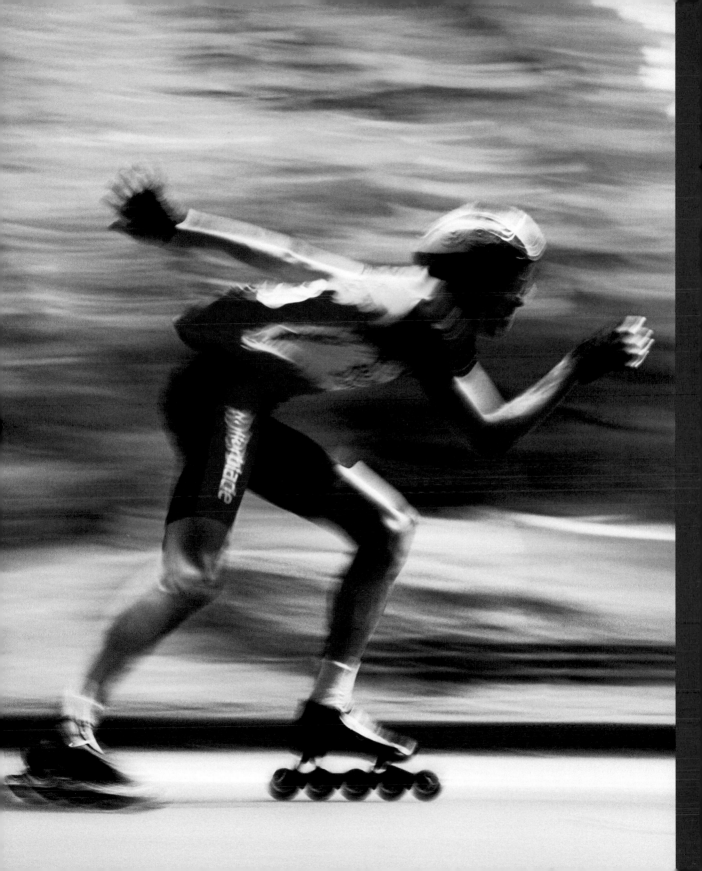

ten-point plan for lifestyle changes at leisure for energy

If you don't have any leisure time, it's your own fault, and if you have it but don't use it properly, that's your own fault too. Don't forget that all work and no play makes Jack a dull and tired boy and in today's world, it's likely to be just as true, if not more true, for Jill as well. Feeling energetic is one of the really good things in life and the good things are worth struggling for.

This ten-point action plan will make the struggle a great deal easier and the prize at the end is worth more than a pot of gold. You'll have a boundless supply of energy which will let you enjoy your leisure to the full.

1 Prioritize your time. Work out a schedule and allocate at least five hours in each working week as private leisure time – and that doesn't include your lunch hour or the time you spend traveling to and from work.

2 At weekends you must set aside at least one continuous three-hour period or two sets of two hours for leisure activities on your own or with friends and family.

3 Use some of your leisure time for relaxation exercises. These will give your mental and emotional energy an immediate boost (see page 110–111). Contrary to popular belief, mental therapies like yoga, meditation, visualization, self-hypnosis, and even prayer, are all great stress-busters, which is why they are so effective. Emotional tension creates anxiety, which triggers excessive production of the hormone adrenaline. This prepares the body for fight or flight, which in turn causes muscle tension. Prolonged periods of this type of stress mean that your muscles are constantly ready for action and permanently in a state of contraction, and this results in pain, discomfort, and the relentless burning up of your energy reserves by all that muscular effort.

4 Make sure you channel some of your leisure time into cultural activities, as these are another key to good mental energy. It makes no difference at all whether your cultural activities consist of going to pop festivals, discos and clubs, or visiting art galleries, listening to chamber music, or going to the opera. It doesn't matter whether you prefer to read sex-and-shopping novels, sci-fi and mysteries, or philosophy, the classics, and historical novels. What is important is satisfying your spiritual need for cultural stimulus.

5 Another great source of mental energy is playing games. This is also a brilliant way of building relationships with friends, family, and children. You must choose a game that's appropriate to your playing companions, but it absolutely doesn't matter whether it's slap jack or bridge, Monopoly or Scrabble, snakes and ladders or tiddlywinks, charades or Trivial Pursuit. Any of these games will shake up the gray matter and, win or lose, will give you a mental-energy boost. Just keep away from the computer and the Game Boy.

6 Now it's time to get physical. I always have problems when I tell patients who suffer from chronic fatigue that they need to take some physical exercise, as it's the last thing they feel like doing. But getting the body moving releases the feelgood hormones in the brain and the energy-packing activity hormones in the rest of the body. No matter how tired you feel when you get home from work, do something physical.

7 Choose appropriate exercise. If you're looking for a burst of super energy on a regular basis, you have to choose a form of activity that is appropriate to your age and general health. If you've been a couch potato for years, don't start with advanced aerobics or long-distance running. Begin slowly and build up to three regular sessions of 20–30 minutes a week. Even a brisk walk – enough to make you sweat and get home slightly out of breath – will start the process off.

8 Choose exercise you enjoy – if you hate it you'll never keep it up. Ideally, try to ensure you do a different type of exercise for each period of leisure time that you set aside. Walking, swimming, and golf would be a great combination. But you can just as well choose tennis, squash, bowling, line dancing, folk dancing, cycling, jogging, or even gardening. Just remember that the object is to generate energy, and this will happen automatically the more you exercise.

9 If you're getting physical, do take sensible precautions. If you decide to use a mini-scooter, roller blades, or a bicycle, then make sure you wear the proper protective gear, as you won't generate much energy lying in a hospital bed with a fractured skull or kneecap.

10 Keep at it. Be committed, be regular, and don't allow outside pressures like work to interfere with your leisure time.

the perils of life in the 24/7 society

Isn't it great? You can shop in the supermarket at two in the morning, go on-line, check your bank balance and pay your bills at three, nip round to the all-night gas station, fill your tank, have a coffee and a doughnut at four and still get home to watch a movie on satellite TV before it's time to pour the milk on your breakfast cereal. An hour's catnap and you're off to work.

Even the Sunday morning sleep-in, followed by a leisurely breakfast with the kids and a family lunch, have vanished. Seventy-eight percent of you are up and doing by nine o'clock, checking your emails, reading your text messages, or answering your cell phone. Then 50 percent of you go shopping and 25 percent go to work – what sort of rest is this?

It's not so long ago that in many countries all shops shut for lunch, had one day a week when they closed in the afternoon, and none stayed open all day on Saturday, let alone open at all on Sunday. Sunday really was a day of rest, when everyone could recharge their batteries. But not any more.

shift workers

Because we inhabit the non-stop world of 24/7 living, far more people now have to work shifts and they're the ones that suffer the worst health problems. Professor Neil Stanley, Chairman of the British Sleep Society, is one of the world's experts on conditions caused by disrupted sleep patterns. "My major concern is accidents," says the professor. "World catastrophes like the Exxon Valdez oil spill, the Chernobyl and Three Mile Island nuclear accidents, and the Bhopal chemical explosion in India, all happened in the small hours of the night shift, when people's concentration, alertness and energy were at their lowest ebb.

"It's well documented that driving home after the night shift makes you more likely to have an accident than if you're four times over the alcohol limit, and you're 40 percent more likely to have any sort of accident, whether it's in the car or at home. There is no doubt that shift work kills you early as well as making you tired."

the effects on women

Everyone suffers the effects of 24/7 living, but women seem to come off worst. Constant disruptions of regular sleep patterns increase the risk of breast cancer and women working a night shift at least once a week for three years or more have a 60 percent increased risk. Being exposed to bright light all through the working night increases estrogen levels, which also upsets the menstrual cycle. This can be the trigger of PMS, irregular periods, and fertility problems, and when women do manage to conceive they're more likely to have difficult pregnancies.

the effects on men

The 24/7 lifestyle affects men, too. According to the British Trades Union Council, when men have to work late into the night, their jobs may put them at greater risk of physical violence. Late-night gas station attendants and small shop, restaurant, or takeout owners and staff are vulnerable when bars and clubs close.

If the men are actually on shift work, their chances of developing serious heart disease go up by a frightening 40 percent and they're far more likely than other male workers to suffer from lack of energy and chronic fatigue. And on top of that, shift workers commonly have constipation and stomach problems due to dehydration, irregular meals, and bad eating habits.

the effects on children

Youngsters aren't immune either. Do you know what your children do once you've gone to bed? Many are on their computers or text-messaging their friends. Play Stations and video and DVD players are in overdrive. No wonder it's difficult to wake your children in the morning and they haven't got the energy to last the day – they've probably only had three or four hours' sleep. They become disruptive at school, neglect their homework, and even fall asleep during classes. Once their regular sleep patterns are disrupted, it's very hard to re-establish them. Then they suffer energy loss and illness just the same as adults.

eating to survive the 24/7 society

Living life on the 24/7 treadmill is similar to being jetlagged, but its results are permanent and they're not going to go away after a few nights' sleep. As your symptoms get worse, you look for crutches and these usually take the form of caffeine and more caffeine, alcohol and more alcohol, cigarettes and more cigarettes. And often, when you finally do decide to go to bed for a few hours, you'll knock back a sleeping pill or two.

So what are you to do? Well, obviously, unless you have to work night shifts – in which case perhaps you should think about changing your job – you need to start by living your life differently and resist the temptation to stay up night after night.

Next, you should follow the detox for energy plans. If your system's become weighed down by fatigue, this will give it the kick-start it needs.

And you should also follow my seven eating tips to help keep your energy levels up to the mark at all times.

▶ Be a grazer. Eat lots of small meals throughout the day (or night) to stoke up your energy. If you don't allow yourself to get hungry, you won't reach for the high-sugar, high-fat snacks that pile on the pounds.

▶ Always carry a bag of mixed dried fruits, nuts, and seeds. They'll give you a mixture of instant and slow-release energy, plus masses of vitamins and minerals.

▶ Eat as wide a variety of foods as you can. It's the easiest thing in the world to eat the same lunchtime sandwich or soup, or to take the same potato to pop in the workplace microwave, but this means that you don't get the spread of essential nutrients that you need.

▶ When winter comes, take a couple of whole-wheat rolls and a thermos of high-energy hot food to work – a home-made vegetable soup, for instance, or a warming casserole or stew. Add some fresh fruit and you've got a really energy-giving, sustaining, and nourishing feast.

▶ Try not to eat at your desk or workstation. If there's a cafeteria, there must be something healthy on the menu. If not, go out for the occasional pizza and salad or for a takeout shish kebab in pita bread.

▶ Pita bread and raw vegetable sticks with hummus or guacamole and a piece of exotic fresh fruit like kiwi, papaya, or mango make an interesting energy-boosting lunchtime variation.

And when you're at work, don't forget to take proper breaks, and get some fresh air and exercise. If the weather's bad, at least find somewhere other than your desk to sit and read a paper or a book. You'll get back to work refreshed and more productive — which should please the boss!

supplementary help

You may have followed the detox program and taken the supplements I suggested, but the following four are worth taking regularly. They're not meant as crutches to keep you going when you shouldn't, but they can help energize you when you need it.

▶ Guarana – the Brazilian rainforest energy herb
▶ Co-enzyme Q – helps the body convert food into energy
▶ Ginseng – the Chinese herb for stamina
▶ Vitamin B complex – essential for the nervous system

kick-start your karma

In strictly chemical terms, energy is the result of combustion. The body uses the food you eat as fuel, the fuel is burned just like the gas in your furnace, and that releases the energy that allows the body to perfom its daily tasks. But this is a very simplistic and mechanistic approach to what really happens. Since the dawn of time, shamans, medicine men, druids, priests, and mystics have understood the immense power of spiritual energy and if you could learn to harness and use it yourself, you'd find a whole new dimension opening in your life. Spiritual energy will give you a reservoir of support that you can draw on whenever you need it. It will be constantly available to give the edge to the performance of whatever task you're undertaking, and you'll find that every problem is easier to resolve.

During my many years in practice, I've seen patients who eat the best possible diet and whose lives are meticulously organized, at home and at work. Yet they lack that vital spark. Life always appears to be an uphill struggle. Conversely, I've seen those who live on burgers and fries and whose lives are chaotic, but they emanate the huge vibrational force of an energetic spirit. They have an aura of stimulating and at the same time comforting and safe energy which envelops those close to them. Wherever they go, they're always the center of attention and the reason is that they have found a way of getting in touch with their spiritual energy.

For many people, religion is the key to tapping into their spiritual energy. You may find it through formal religious belief and observance or by the loosest association with ancient mystical ideals. But it doesn't matter how you reach your goal. It's a question of what suits you best and often your personal cultural background points you in the right direction.

People tend to believe that it's only the ancient eastern religions that can take you along the path to enlightenment, but this isn't true. Certainly the traditions of the East like yoga, meditation, and deep relaxation are all excellent ways to develop energy-building spiritual insights, but contrary to some misinformed opinions, it's not necessary to embrace eastern religious beliefs in order to get the benefits of meditation. You simply have to learn the physical skills necessary in order to focus your mind and concentrate on attaining a state of heightened spiritual awareness. And like all physical skills, it's simply a question of a good teacher and lots of practice.

Other people tap into their spiritual energy through ancient earth-based practices, with their incantations and group religious ceremonies, while yet others choose a more mechanistic art, such as feng shui. Sadly, feng shui has been adopted in recent years by interior designers and so has become debased, but in fact, it's an integral part of the whole philosophy of traditional acupuncture and is dependent on a balance of yin and yang to create sensations of perfect harmony. These, in turn, bring spiritual awareness and spiritual energy.

Christianity has much to offer, too, not only for the profound beliefs it sets out, but also in terms of ritual. Using the rosary for a Catholic, contemplating icons in the Greek or Russian orthodox churches, the rituals of communion, the repetitive phrases of plainsong chant – these have exactly the same effect as Bhuddist chanting or repeating your mantra before you meditate. They're all just different ways of reaching the same goal.

I know many people whose lives have literally been turned around once they've overcome their prejudices and allowed themselves to believe that vital energy and real health come from the holistic trilogy of mind, body, and spirit. But for some, this is an uncomfortable place to go. I recommend you try it – you've nothing to lose. You don't have to embrace a new religion, there is no need to give up whatever you already believe in. It can't do you any harm and for those who persevere, the rewards can be truly amazing.

shortcut to nirvana

As I've already said, relaxation exercises give your mental and emotional energy an immediate boost. This simple exercise slows the heartbeat and the breathing rate and will refresh and renew you. To begin with, you'll need about half an hour, but as you become practiced, you'll reach the ideal state of mental and physical relaxation in less time.

▶ Choose a warm room, turn off the radio or television, disconnect the telephone and lie flat on a very firm bed or on a rug on the floor. Try to empty your mind of thoughts and emotions.

▶ Close your eyes and take three deep, slow breaths in and out.

▶ Stretch your left leg along the floor away from your body as hard as you can, pointing your foot and contracting the calf, thigh, buttock, and lower back muscles. Hold that position until you feel a slight trembling in the muscles, then relax. Repeat with the right leg; then with both legs, and relax again.

▶ Stretch your left arm down your side, spreading your fingers and pushing from the big muscles at the back of the neck and shoulder so that you contract all the muscles of the upper arm, forearm, and hand. Relax.

▶ Repeat with the right arm and relax. Repeat with both arms and relax again.

▶ Stretch both arms and legs together and relax.

▶ Take five deep breaths and repeat the cycle again. Repeat the cycle four more times.

▶ Relax totally for 10 minutes, preferably with a blanket within reach, as your body temperature may drop as a result of your slower heart beat and lower breathing rates.

the benefits of relaxation

Once you're relaxed, a number of physical and physiological changes occur within your body. You'll feel a sensation of heaviness together with a sense of clearer perception and heightened awareness. Your pulse rate will go down and because your heart is pumping more slowly, you'll be aware that your entire system seems to be slowing down too. One of the damaging effects of stress is that the levels of sugar and fat circulating in your bloodstream increase. As you become more practiced at controling your stress levels through relaxation, these levels will drop.

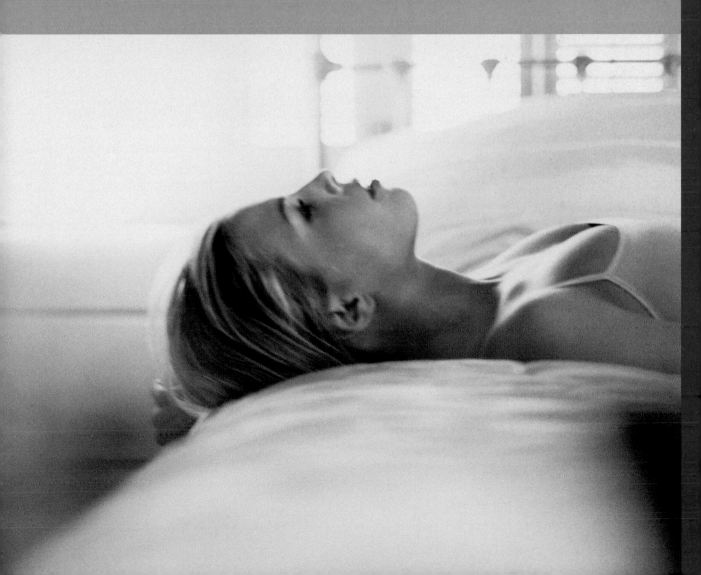

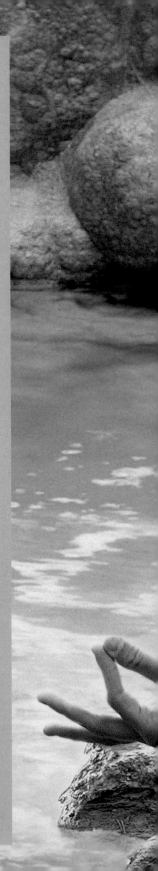

meditation

Meditation has been used for thousands of years. Its purpose is the search for the harmonization of the way things are – reality – and the way they should be – the ideal. When you meditate, you reach a state of awareness where your mind is emptied of everything. You experience a state of restful alertness and mental and spiritual energy.

The main components of meditation are:

- a clearer understanding and appreciation of the ideal order of things through enhanced awareness
- development of an open mind that will be receptive to reality
- to be spiritually and physically active in translating the ideal to reality.

The practice of meditation in the west has tended to put greatest emphasis on the understanding and appreciation of the ideal. This is visualized during periods of silent contemplation and restful alertness. To reach this state, you must focus all your concentration on a single object and to help you do this, you may constantly repeat a word or phrase, traditionally known as a mantra. This rhythmic chanting, with its hypnotic and vibrational effects, produces a trance-like state that leads your body and mind into the meditative state. It is this that produces the extraordinary health benefits. As well as producing an explosion of mental energy, regular meditation dramatically reduces your risks of heart disease, high blood pressure, and strokes, and also helps combat tension, anxiety, and stress-related diseases.

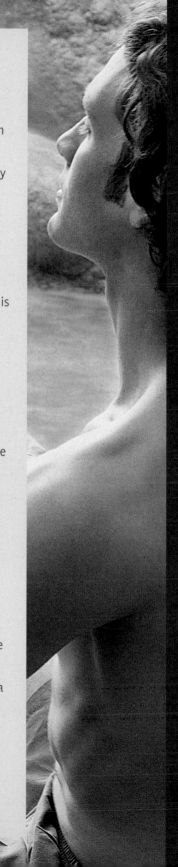

a simple guide to meditation

Over the years I've been regularly amazed at the inner peace and calm, together with the vibrant energy that I've seen in practicing Buddhists and others who use meditation in their everyday lives. Experience has taught me that to become seriously involved in meditation takes time, dedication, and commitment, which not all of us are lucky enough to have. For this reason, I've devised a simplified scheme to encourage people to dip their toe into the water of this intensely spiritual practice.

If you persevere, I'm certain that you will gain so much from meditation that you'll want to understand it better and look further into its deeper meaning. Here, though, is where to start.

▶ Get into a comfortable position. It doesn't matter if you sit, lie, or recline, as long as the radio and television are off, and you've unplugged the telephone.
▶ Close your eyes.
▶ Work your way through the Short Cut to Nirvana program (see pages 110–111).
▶ Breathe in deeply through your nose and out through your mouth, at the same time trying to empty your mind of all thoughts. While doing this, repeat your chosen mantra – the word "one" is widely used – preferably out loud and as deeply in your voice register as you can, as this helps to create the vibration.
▶ Continue breathing deeply and evenly for at least 10 or preferably 20 minutes. Keep pushing away any distracting thoughts while constantly repeating the mantra.
▶ When you've finished, remain completely still with your eyes closed for 2–3 minutes, then open your eyes but stay where you are for another minute or two.

Deep meditation can often trigger unexpected results. Most commonly, these take the form of sudden uncontrolled emotional outbursts like laughing or crying. If this happens to you, don't worry. It's quite normal. In fact, you should be pleased as it's a sign that you really have reached a deep state of relaxation.

mind games

You've energized your body with a detox and with exercise, but your mind needs energizing as well. In fact, the old adage "use it or lose it" is just as applicable to mental processes as it is to your back, leg, or any other muscles.

Of course you use your mind all day long as you make minute-to-minute decisions – you use it when you cook, shop, drive your car, even to make sure you get on the right bus. But these are hardly intellectually demanding activities and they don't stretch your mental powers.

To really generate revitalizing mental energy you have to make your brain cells work, and work hard at that. You'll only achieve this by constantly challenging your mental abilities and always seeking to push a little beyond what you think you can achieve.

improving short-term memory

Maintaining and improving short-term memory is fundamental to exercising your mental functions and allowing you to access your huge reserves of mental energy. Nothing burns up mental energy more than constantly searching through your mind for that elusive word, name, date, or telephone number. Although short-term memory tends to decrease with age, it's frequently a problem of young people as well. As long as you're not suffering from any severe deterioration in brain function, every one of you should be able to sharpen up your memory and speed the access to your brain's databanks. Try the following:

▶ Kim's Game – an old stand-by of the worldwide Boy Scout movement – is one of the great memory improvers. Have someone place 20 different objects on a tray, cover it with a cloth and then allow you to look at the objects for 60 seconds. Replace the cloth, then try tp write down as many objects as you can remember. Initially you may struggle to remember more than a handful, but with regular practice you'll be amazed at how quickly you'll be able to recall almost all of them.

▶ Learning by heart – you can improve both short- and long-term memory by learning poetry, speeches from plays, or quotations from well-known books. To make this work, you have to do it on a regular basis, so every night before you go to bed, commit a few lines to memory and make sure you can repeat them the next morning, and the morning after that, and a month after that. You may not have tried to memorize a poem since your schooldays, but the mental energy it generates will mean a permanent improvement. You may find you can't manage more than five or six lines to begin with, but before you know it, your party piece will be the opening prologue from Shakespeare's Henry V.

exercise those brain cells

Another really effective way to prevent a decline in your short-term memory function is to practice mental arithmetic for a few minutes every single day. Try these mental math exercises. The answers are on page 256.

1. $10 \times 10 + 12$

2. $\dfrac{7 \times 8 \times 2 - 2}{10}$

3. $\dfrac{13 + 7}{5 \times 12}$

4. $\dfrac{23 \times 4 - 50}{7}$

5. $17 + 14 + 106 + 33 - 27$

6. $109 + 72 + 226 + 593$

7. $10{,}425 + 8{,}659 + 28{,}694 \times 100$

Anagrams

1. PARTIAL MEN
2. OLD WEST ACTION
3. GENTLEMAN RYE
4. DE PEG SURREY EX NOT
5. DUESOX
6. BEG FREE RUB
7. IMBO RIN GRANTS

beat the sugar trap

Have you ever eaten a couple of cookies, a bowl of cornflakes or a chocolate bar? I bet you have. If so, you may have noticed how, a little while later, you feel full of pep and a few hours after that, you're jittery, unable to concentrate and dying for a little sugary fix. This is because you're now suffering – if only in passing – from hypoglycemia or low blood sugar. It's sometimes called the "Sugar Blues."

When carbohydrate foods are eaten, the sugars they contain are broken down into glucose during digestion. Glucose – or blood sugar as it is also confusingly known – is the fuel our bodies run on. The glucose circulating in our bloodstream after a carbohydrate meal is circulated to cells for instant use, and any surplus is converted into glycogen and stored as fuel in the liver, ready to be "switched on" whenever it is needed. The hormone insulin, secreted by the pancreas, is responsible for this storage job.

Eat a slice of whole-grain bread, a dish of lentils, or a handful of ripe apricots, and the sugars in them are broken down into glucose quite slowly. But when you eat your cookies, cornflakes, or chocolate – known as high-glycemic foods – the sugars they contain will be broken down very quickly, sending the glucose level in your bloodstream rocketing.

The pancreas responds to this abnormal situation by pumping out extra insulin, so your blood-sugar levels drop sharply – giving you the "Sugar Blues."

The sugar in processed food – aided and abetted by the food-manufacturing industry – is obviously the real villain of the piece and it's hard to avoid. It's there in desserts, juices, canned drinks, sugar-coated breakfast cereals, cookies, ice cream, snacks, and sweets. Once you've acquired a sweet tooth, it's not long before every cup of tea or coffee needs three heaped spoons of sugar and every unoccupied moment is filled with a cookie, a piece of cake, or a Danish pastry.

the effects on your health

The fluctuations in blood-sugar levels caused by eating these foods have been linked with a huge spectrum of health problems. Long term, they will be responsible for high blood pressure, obesity, diabetes, and heart disease. In children they may be responsible for disruptive behavior, hyperactivity, and an inability to concentrate. And one of the commonest symptoms of low blood sugar is mental and physical fatigue – which may account for the state of permanent exhaustion that is suffered by so many adults, teenagers, and children.

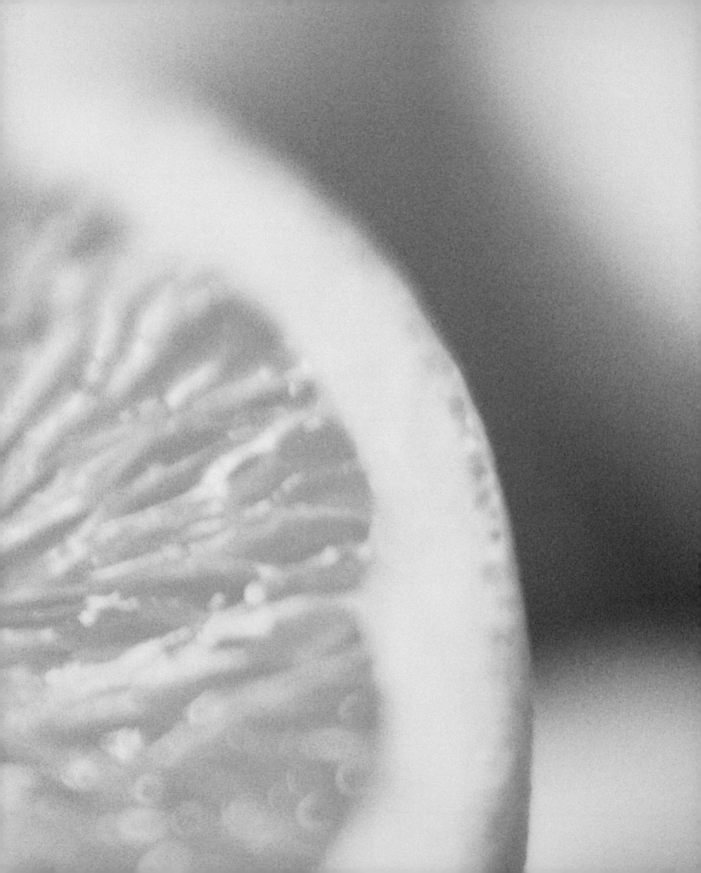

the glycemic index

The glycemic index – GI – is a way of calculating the rate at which carbohydrate foods are digested and converted into sugar by the body. The lower a food's GI, the longer it takes for that food to be converted into sugar. Using the GI can be a great help in planning a healthy diet that will provide you with a gradual release of energy and so help you avoid the sugar trap. By mixing low GI foods into a meal, you'll be able to maintain a much more even level of blood sugar and so ensure a constant flow of mental and physical energy.

Taking 100 as the standard, processed foods like white bread, sugared breakfast cereals, puffed rice, cornflakes, puffed wheat, cookies, instant mashed potato, corn chips, glucose, and honey, all have a GI between 70 and 100. Foods with a GI below 60 are whole wheat, rye and pumpernickel, whole-wheat pasta, brown rice, corn, buckwheat, bulgur, wholewheat kernels, whole rye kernels, pearl barley, shredded wheat, oatmeal, chickpeas, soy beans, all dried beans, and low-fat dairy foods.

other processed-food problems

While we all need plenty of carbohydrate foods to give us physical as well as mental energy, the best of them supply more than just energy. Foods such as whole-grain bread, brown rice, whole oats, beans and lentils and fruits are also loaded with important nutrients and are rich in fiber, which helps keep the digestive system functioning efficiently. But when these foods are refined or heavily processed, they lose not only a whole slew of vital nutrients, but most of the fiber too.

To take just one example, white flour contains much less zinc (essential for resistance, mental energy, and male sexual function), much less magnesium (vital for the nervous system and also for the absorption of calcium), and significantly less protein (essential for body-building) than whole-wheat flour. Token amounts of major nutrients are added back when white flour is baked into bread, but not when it goes into other foods.

It's the same story when rice and corn are refined. And white sugar has absolutely no nutritional value at all, except for a lot of energy-giving calories – styled "empty" calories for this very reason. Brown sugar and honey at least contain traces of key nutrients.

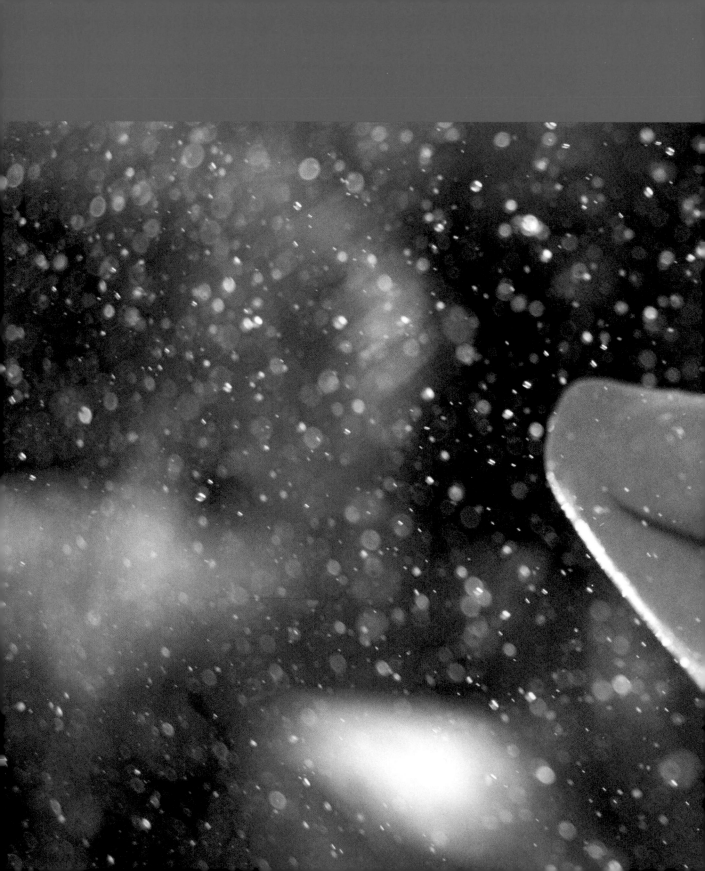

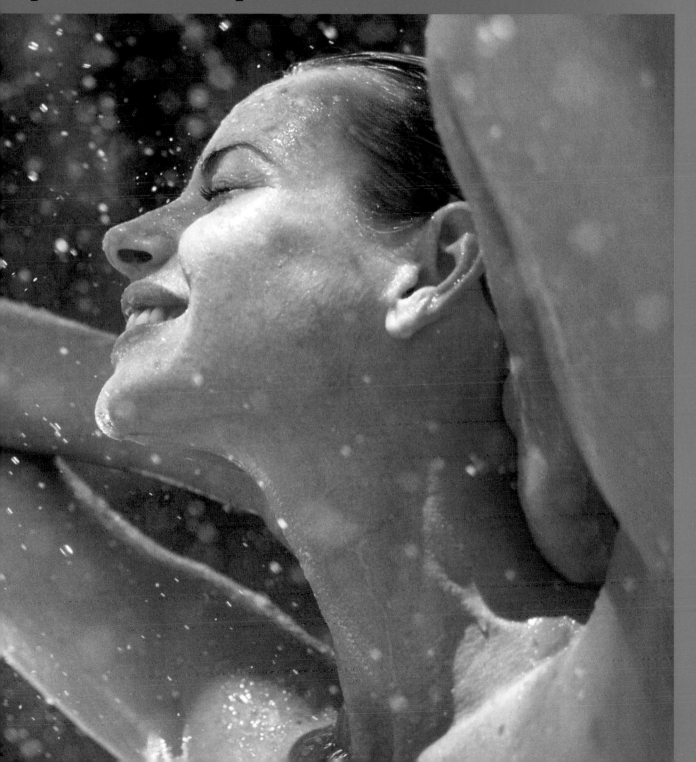

part 3 super radiance detox

the search for super radiance

"It looks good, tastes good and by golly it does you good" may be one of the great advertising slogans of all time, but there's a lot of truth in it, just as there is in the saying "You are what you eat." This is especially the case when it comes to radiance.

People imagine that to be radiant, you have to be young and beautiful, but this is far from the truth. Radiance has nothing to do with the conventional perception of "beauty." No-one could describe Mrs. Ghandi, the late prime minister of India, as a beauty, but I sat next to her once at a small private dinner and she positively oozed radiance.

The truth is that to look radiant on the outside you have to be radiant on the inside. It's the combination of both that results in super radiance. It shows in healthy skin, hair, and nails, but it comes from general good health, good bowel function, strong bones, and pain-free joints, and you can achieve all these by eating the right things and clearing all the rubbish out of your system.

So if you've looked in the mirror and think you're sliding down the radiance scale, now's the time to take control, start your detox for radiance plan, and change your eating habits for good. Simple changes can not only stop the clock, but can even turn it back.

If your idea of cooking is ready meals from the freezer to the microwave, instant soups, noodles, and takeout food, then you shouldn't be surprised if your skin looks less than radiant. People forget that skin is one of the body's major organs of elimination, and many of the waste products and irritant materials that result from the chemical factory that makes up your daily metabolism find their way to the outside world through this delicate membrane. Efficient elimination of bodily waste will also be hampered by constipation, which is a frequent cause of dull and lifeless skin. It's also uncomfortable and can produce painful gas and unsightly bloating, which in turn makes it difficult to wear any clothes that fit snugly around the waist. Proper detoxing and long-term changes to your eating patterns can solve even a lifetime of constipation and will enable you to live without the bowel-irritating effects of laxatives.

Excessive amounts of alcohol and caffeine may also be implicated as the cause of some skin problems. These are both vasoconstrictors – they narrow the tiny blood capillaries at the end of the circulatory system – and can restrict the flow of vital nutrients to the skin.

In addition, protecting your joints, ligaments, and muscles is a must, as there is nothing as certain as pain to dull your natural radiance. Similarly, you need protection from degenerative diseases like arthritis and osteoporosis, and to ward off heart disease, strokes, and cancer. Again, what you eat has a bearing on all of this, and once you have gotten into the regular habit of detoxing to keep the chemical load to a minimum, you must restructure your everyday eating to include all of the most essential foods.

And finally, don't forget that environmental pollution, pregnancy, stress, anxiety, depression, menstruation, thyroid problems, menopause and, of course, smoking, can all play their part in denying you the radiance you deserve.

time to detox?

Dull blotchy skin, lifeless hair, breaking fingernails, early wrinkles, cellulite, and a total absence of radiance can be the result of poor nutrition, external toxic damage from too much sun, smoking, and environmental pollution, or an internal accumulation of waste products. Your radiance can also be affected by too much booze. This is not only damaging on its own, but also interferes with your body's ability to absorb nutrients. Any chronic digestive disease can also do this and thyroid problems, long-term illness, pain, and the side effects of medication can all be equally damaging. Answer the Super Radiance quiz now to learn just how much you need to start the regime.

1 How many times a week do you eat yellow, red or orange fruits and vegetables?
- **A** Every day.
- **B** Most days.
- **C** Hardly ever.

2 How many times a week do you eat dark green leafy vegetables?
- **A** Every day.
- **B** Most days.
- **C** Hardly ever.

3 How often do you eat processed foods like lunch meat, frozen entrees, and sausage?
- **A** Never – I love cooking proper meals.
- **B** Rarely – but I do eat them three or four times a week when I'm busy.
- **C** Most of the time – they're so much easier than having to cook.

4 What type of oil or fat do you use for cooking?
- **A** Olive oil – the best extra-virgin, organic brand I can afford.
- **B** Sunflower, canola or other seed oil.
- **C** Butter, lard, hard margarine, or anything else that's lurking in the fridge.

5 Do you eat oily fish like salmon, sardines, or mackerel?
- **A** Yes, at least once a week – I know it's good for me.
- **B** Occasionally – but I know I should eat more.
- **C** Oily fish? What's that?

6 How much water do you drink a day?
- **A** More than 6 glasses.
- **B** 3–6 glasses.
- **C** 2 or less.

7 How many cups of coffee do you drink each day?
- **A** 3 or less.
- **B** 3–6.
- **C** More than 6.

8 Do you (check as many as you like)
Smoke
Drink more than 14 drinks (women) or 21 drinks (men) of alcohol a week

Take sleeping pills/tranquilizers/anti-depressants
Use recreational drugs

9 How important is exercise to you?

   A Very – I go jogging nearly every day.

   B Quite important – I probably do half an hour or so three or four times a week.

   C Not important at all – I've never been sporty and I don't intend to start now!

10 How often do you make time to thoroughly clean and moisturize your skin?

   A Every day.

   B At least three times a week.

   C When I get round to it.

11 Is constipation a problem for you?

   A Never.

   B Occasionally.

   C It has been for years.

12 Do you suffer with an underactive thyroid?

   A No, I've never had a problem.

   B I've had a slight problem but don't take any medication.

   C Yes, I have to take medication every day.

13 Do you have a skin condition which means you have to use steroid creams?

   A No.

   B Occasionally.

   C All the time.

14 Do you take the contraceptive pill or HRT?

   A No.

   B I used to but I've stopped.

   C Yes.

15 How stressful do you consider your life/work to be?

   A Not very.

   B Occasionally when I'm under pressure at home or work.

   C Very, all the time.

Score:

A – 1 point
B – 3 points
C or check – 5 points

Over 85 – start detoxing now. If you're under 20 you can probably get away with your lifestyle and eating habits but, like Dorian Gray, the day will come when everything turns to dust and your radiance will be gone for good. Once you've worked your way through the radiance detox, you must then include as many as possible of the protective foods I recommend in your regular diet.

60–85 – all is not lost. A few changes to your eating and lifestyle, a bit more routine skin care and you'll soon be more radiant than ever before. Pay special attention to the Replenishing for Radiance plan (pages 138–143).

35–60 – you're doing a great job. You're probably eating well, taking care of your skin, enjoying work and home and have very few problems with wrinkles or cellulite.

15–35 – you may be looking great, but I suspect your life is boring. Beauty is more than skin deep.

cleansing for

Radiance is difficult to measure and even harder to describe, but we all know it when we see it. Bad hair days, lackluster eyes, and sallow skin don't make anyone look very radiant. No detox regime is going to make up for years of smoking, drinking, and burning the candle at both ends, so if these habits are the cause of your lack of radiance, they must be tackled now.

But if you're young and willing, you can boost and maintain your natural youthful radiance with appropriate detoxing. Even if you're not so young and the first flush of youth has passed you by, it's not too late. Your skin is a remarkable organ and totally replaces itself with a new layer roughly every six weeks, so you still have a chance to rekindle your radiance.

when should I detox?

Regular twenty-four hour juice fasts are a powerful weapon in the defense of your radiance and even if you have unblemished skin, it's great to follow the twenty-four hour plan at least once a month. Extend it to the forty-eight hour plan in extraordinary situations, for example after indulging in too much Easter candy, or when you're having an extra stressful time at work. Four times a year, to coincide with the seasons, you should do the full three-day detox as a radiance renewing exercise. It's particularly effective after Christmas and in early spring to make up for over-indulgence, bad weather, and lack of sunshine. And if you repeat it in late summer and again in late autumn, it will pump your system full of protective anti-oxidants that help give you a healthy glow throughout the winter months. If you need to fast for therapeutic reasons, to restore your radiance after illness, injury, or periods of severe stress, then the three-day program is again ideal.

radiance

The twenty-four and forty-eight hour plans are real fasts. The twenty-four hour fast includes no solid food at all, and the forty-eight hour one very little – just some fresh and dried fruit and some nuts. The three-day program introduces yogurt, cooked vegetables, a soup, and pasta. This fast is certainly not suitable to do while you're working, as you need at least one day to recover before going back to your normal activities.

side effects

You're bound to have some side effects, but don't worry. They're a sign the detox is working. The most common side effect is a headache – this can happen even on a twenty-four hour program. On a forty-eight hour or three-day detox you may also experience a "healing crisis" – increased temperature, sweating, tremors, and general aches and pains. For detailed information on these side effects and how to manage them, see page 13.

take care

If you suffer with any health problems, always consult your regular physician before starting a detox program. And it's really important to take my advice on the supplements you need (see pages 128–129).

the extras

Please don't start any of the plans without being fully prepared. Read through them in detail and make sure you stock up on the foods and supplements that you're going to need, as there's nothing more frustrating than getting ready mentally, putting up with the first day, and then not being able to complete your detox as effectively as possible.

what to drink

I recommend that first thing in the morning you make up a pitcher of Parsley Tea (see recipe, page 189). Keep it in the fridge and drink small glasses regularly throughout the day. This gentle diuretic will help to speed up the detoxifying and cleansing processes, so make sure you drink it all.

While you can drink as much water, herb, or weak green tea as you like, you shouldn't add milk or any sweetening. And you mustn't consume fizzy water, canned drinks, alcohol, black tea, coffee, or any sweetened drinks. This includes sugar-free commercial drinks, which contain artificial sweeteners instead.

the supplements

With any detox program, whether it's the twenty-four-hour detox, the forty-eight-hour detox, the three-day detox, or the eight-day return to normal, you can improve the efficiency of the plan and support your body's system throughout the program by using the appropriate supplements every day.

for general well-being

When you're following these programs, you'll be eating much less food than usual. The recommended foods provide an abundance of nutrients; nevertheless, it's important to give the body an extra boost of vitamins and minerals to avoid any possible deficiencies and to guarantee optimum levels. For this reason you should take:

▶ A high-potency multi-vitamin and mineral supplement (choose one of the reputable brand leaders)

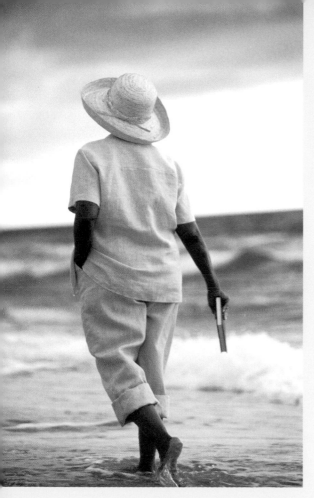

▶ 500mg vitamin C, three times a day. If you can find it, use ester-C, which many leading manufacturers are now including in their products as it is non-acidic and less likely to cause digestive upsets, especially while you're eating less food

▶ A one-a-day standardized extract of cynarin – from globe artichokes. Cynarin stimulates liver function and helps the body to eliminate the many fat-soluble substances that are stored in the liver.

for bowel function

Maintaining proper and regular bowel function is always important but especially when you are detoxing.

▶ To stimulate, improve, and maintain bowel function take 1–2 tablespoons of oatbran or ground psyllium seed every night while you follow the plans and, for best results, start the day before. Both provide water-soluble fiber – better described as smoothage rather than roughage.

for all-around radiance

▶ A supplement of selenium with vitamins A, C, and E
▶ A supplement of betacarotene, lutein, zeaxanthine, and other carotenoids
▶ A probiotic supplement of gut-friendly bacteria.

for specific radiance problems

▶ Ginkgo biloba for thread veins, varicose veins, and poor peripheral circulation
▶ Evening primrose oil for dry scaly skin and eczema
▶ Magnesium for nail problems
▶ Silica and saw palmetto for thinning hair.

rest and exercise

While you're following the detox programs, get a little extra rest but also take two or three short walks – not more than 10–15 minutes – each day. Don't jog, run, go to the gym, or do strenuous jobs around the house and yard, as over-exertion will drain your energy, produce toxic chemical by-products, and inhibit your cleansing regime.

twenty-four hour cleansing

Whether you use this twenty-four-hour Cleansing for Radiance fast as a regular radiance boost or feel you need it because you've just had a weekend of rich food and too much alcohol, you'll find it's really worth the effort – just take a look in the mirror twenty-four hours later to see the difference.

It's a short sharp treatment that anyone can fit into a busy life. You'll be more comfortable if you do it when you're not working, but most people in reasonable health can manage these twenty-four hours without taking time off.

on waking   A large glass of hot water with a thick slice of organic unwaxed lemon

breakfast   A large glass of hot water with a thick slice of organic unwaxed lemon
A glass of Radiance Juice (see recipe, page 190)
A mug of nettle tea

mid-morning   A large glass of hot water with a thick slice of organic unwaxed lemon

lunch   A large glass of Tomato Juice with Garlic and Green Onions (see recipe, page 187)
A mug of nettle tea

mid-afternoon   A large glass of hot water with a thick slice of organic unwaxed lemon

supper   Mango, Kiwi, and Pineapple Juice (see recipe, page 191)
A mug of nettle tea

evening   Carrot and Beet Juice (see recipe, page 191)

bedtime   A mug of lime-blossom (linden or tilia) tea

forty-eight hour cleansing

Start by following the twenty-four hour Cleansing for Radiance plan, then have:

on waking A large glass of hot water with a thick slice of organic unwaxed lemon

breakfast A large glass of hot water with a thick slice of organic unwaxed lemon
A large glass of Radiance Juice (see recipe, page 190)
A mug of nettle tea

mid-morning A large glass of hot water with a thick slice of organic unwaxed lemon

lunch A glass of Radiance Lemonade (see recipe, page 190)
A mug of mint tea

mid-afternoon A large glass of hot water with a thick slice of organic unwaxed lemon

supper A large bowl of fresh fruit salad, to include apple, pear, grapes, mango, and some berries
– but no banana
A handful of raisins – chew them very slowly – and a handful of fresh, unsalted
cashew nuts
A mug of mint tea

evening A large glass of hot water with a thick slice of organic unwaxed lemon

bedtime A mug of camomile tea with a teaspoon of organic honey

three-day cleansing

You may already have tried the twenty-four or forty-eight hour fasts and I'm sure you were surprised at how easy they were. Now it's time for you to graduate into the "grown-ups" league. When you wake up on day 4 your body will feel lighter, your system cleaner, and your eyes and skin will have a sparkle and luster you haven't seen in ages. You'll also be overflowing with all the protective anti-oxidants you need and you'll almost certainly have lost over 2 pounds in weight.

These three days are pretty low in calories, providing around 3,000 altogether when your normal intake should be 2,000 a day for women and 3,000 for men. You'll feel hungry from time to time, but don't spoil it by cheating. To help overcome the hunger pangs take two teaspoons of the Swiss herbal tonic BioStrath Elixir, three times a day.

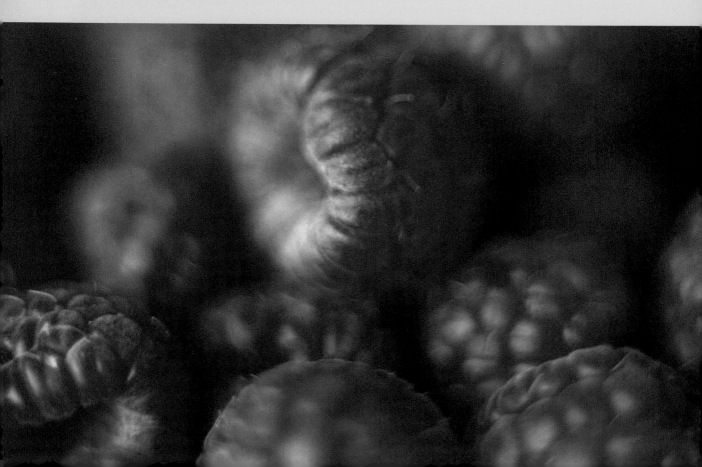

Days 1 and 2, follow the Forty-Eight Hour Cleansing program. Day 3:

on waking   A large glass of hot water with a thick slice of organic unwaxed lemon

breakfast   A large glass of hot water with a thick slice of organic unwaxed lemon
Fresh fruit salad – a mixture of any of the following: apple, pear, grapes, mango, and pineapple and any berries with a carton of live yogurt and a tablespoon of unsweetened muesli.
A cup of weak black tea or herb tea

mid-morning   6 dried apricots
A glass of fruit or vegetable juice

lunch   Chilled Watercress Soup (see recipe, page 235) with a chunk of crusty whole-wheat bread, no butter
A cup of weak black tea or herb tea

mid-afternoon   An apple and a pear

supper   Zucchini Pasta (see recipe, page 217)
A salad of tomato, onion, and yellow bell pepper
A cup of weak black tea or herb tea

eight-day return to normal eating

If you're determined to enjoy the long-term radiance benefits that you've already started to build up, then it's really important to go straight on to the return to normal eating program. Your radiance detox has already started the cleansing process, but this is your opportunity to boost your intake of the super-nutrients that your skin, hair, and nails require to be in optimum condition. This part of the regime also encourages you into a healthier style of eating which reduces your consumption of the anti-radiance foods, especially those that have a high content of damaging free radicals.

As in all the detox plans, you'll be getting plenty of water to stimulate kidney function and waste elimination – both vital for a clear and radiant skin. The powerful anti-oxidant dark-colored berries also feature heavily as they're not only highly protective, but also slow the skin-aging process and help prevent wrinkles. The plan also gives you lots of vegetable juices rich in the minerals that you need for healthy hair and nails. Probiotic foods like live yogurt will give you calcium to protect your bones as well as gut-friendly bacteria, which stimulate your immune system and protect against all types of infections, including fungal and bacterial infections of the scalp, nails, and skin. You'll also enjoy a wide range of culinary herbs, included for their medicinal value as much as for their flavor. Sage, for example, helps even out hormonal irregularities which can have such a debilitating effect on both skin and hair, and which are often a key factor in the cyclical upsets in your overall radiance.

This is a week of no animal protein and even if you're the most dedicated carnivore, don't cheat. Saturated animal fat is not only a hazard to your heart, blood circulation, and blood pressure, it can do severe damage to your radiance. It's a source of free radicals, which attack your body's cells, and it can increase the amount of sebum produced by your skin. The result? Your skin will be greasy and more liable to blocked pores and infected pimples.

It's important that you follow day 1 exactly. The following days are more flexible and you may switch light meals and main meals within (but not between) days.

keeping up your fluid intake

As always, you must keep your fluid intake up to a minimum of one and a half quarts a day, and avoid canned drinks and commercial juices, just as in the detox plans. Once you are in the habit of starting your day with hot water and lemon, you may well find you want to continue with it as part of your normal routine.

Throughout this week take a good quality multi-vitamin and mineral supplement together with a teaspoon of the Swiss Herbal BioStrath Elixir three times a day.

day 1

This is a very special day when your main food will be rice. Like fasting, rice days are traditionally used by naturopaths as a cleansing treatment. Start by preparing the rice for the whole day. You'll need $^3/_4$ cup dry brown rice cooked in 2 cups of water. If you prefer, cook half the rice in half the water, and the other half in vegetable stock for a more savory flavor.

breakfast $^1/_2$ cup cooked rice with $^2/_3$ cup stewed pears flavored with honey, cloves, and lime juice
A large glass of hot water with a thick slice of organic unwaxed lemon

mid-morning A large glass of hot water with a thick slice of organic unwaxed lemon

lunch $^1/_2$ cup cooked rice with $1^1/_2$ cups steamed vegetables — celery, thin slices of red and green bell pepper — tomato purée, garlic, and a drizzle of extra-virgin olive oil
A large glass of hot water with a thick slice of organic unwaxed lemon

mid-afternoon A large glass of hot water with a thick slice of organic unwaxed lemon

supper $^1/_2$ cup cooked rice mixed with yogurt, strawberries, blueberries, banana, and kiwi, all whizzed in a blender
A large glass of hot water with a thick slice of organic unwaxed lemon

bedtime A mug of camomile tea with a teaspoon of organic honey

day 2

breakfast   An orange, half a grapefruit and a large slice of melon
A glass of unsalted vegetable juice and a mug of herb tea

light meal   A plateful of raw red and yellow bell peppers, cucumber, tomato, broccoli, cauliflower, celery, carrots, radishes, and lots of fresh parsley, with extra-virgin olive oil and lemon juice
A large glass of unsweetened fruit juice

main meal   A large salad of lettuce, tomato, watercress, onion, garlic, beets, celeriac, fresh mint, and any herbs you like, with extra-virgin olive oil and lemon juice
A large glass of unsweetened fruit juice or unsalted vegetable juice

day 3

breakfast   Sliced blood oranges and pink grapefruit
A helping of low-fat live yogurt, with a teaspoon each of chopped nuts and honey

light meal   Scrambled eggs and mushrooms
Spiced Apricots (make enough for 3 meals) (see recipe, page 248)

main meal   Stuffed Green Bell Peppers (see recipe, page 217)
A large ripe papaya

day 4

breakfast   Spiced Apricots from day 3 with low-fat live yogurt and an orange

light meal   Potato Cake with Broccoli (see recipe, page 215)

main meal   Tofu, Vegetable, and Cashew Nut Stir-Fry (see recipe, page 218)
Apricot and Almond Crumble (see recipe, page 249)

day 5

breakfast   2 hot whole-wheat rolls with a little butter, and a banana

light meal   Risotto con Salsa Cruda (see recipe, page 221)

main meal Eggplant Caviar with Crudités (see recipe, page 244)
Non-Meatballs in Tomato Sauce (see recipe, page 213)

day 6
breakfast Spiced Apricots from day 3 with low-fat yogurt

light meal Half an avocado, sliced, with watercress, tomatoes, and cucumber on mixed leaves with a generous squeeze of lemon juice
A crusty whole-wheat roll

main meal Cold Beet and Apple Soup (see recipe, page 232)
Quick Chickpea Hot Pot (see recipe, page 215)

day 7
breakfast An orange, an apple, and a banana
Low-fat live yogurt

light meal Salad Vegeçoise (see recipe, page 245)

main meal Lentil and Barley Pilaf (see recipe, page 216)
Pink Grapefruit Sorbet (see recipe, page 251)

day 8
breakfast A large glass of half-orange and half-grapefruit juice
Cold Spiced Baked Apple (see recipe, page 246) with low-fat live yogurt, a tablespoon of oats, and 3 brazil nuts

light meal Zucchini Pasta (see recipe, page 217)

main meal Sage Burgers (see recipe, page 222)
Orange Soufflé Omelette (see recipe, page 250)

replenishing

Knowing what nutrient-containing foods to eat is crucial when it comes to replenishing and maintaining your radiance. To make sure, eat a good selection from all these foods regularly.

vitamin A

This is essential for healing skin damage. Eat a portion of liver (not if you're pregnant), carrots, spinach, broccoli, sweet potato, cantaloupe, nectarines, or dried apricots every day.

vitamin E

A super-radiance nutrient that's important for healthy skin and as a protective anti-oxidant. Get your daily requirements from avocados, asparagus, extra-virgin olive oil, cod-liver oil, wheatgerm oil, sunflower seeds, and almonds.

B vitamins

These are essential, especially for the nervous system, while vitamin B12 also prevents pernicious anemia. The B vitamins are found in yeast, whole-grain cereals, liver, and all meat, and B12 is also in eggs, cheese, yogurt, yeast extracts, and beer.

folic acid

A vital B vitamin that prevents birth defects and heart disease. Meet your daily needs with $3\frac{1}{2}$ ounces of spinach, or 6 ounces of potatoes, chickpeas, broccoli, kale, or asparagus.

vitamin D

This is essential for bone strength, and oily fish, margarine, and eggs are the most important sources – $1\frac{1}{2}$ ounces of herring or kipper, 2 ounces of mackerel, 3 ounces of canned salmon or 5 ounces of canned sardines will all provide your daily requirement.

for radiance

zinc

Vital for healthy skin, make sure you get your full complement of zinc by adding red meat, shellfish, sardines, poultry, kidney beans, and pumpkin seeds to your shopping list.

calcium

This is essential for bones. Find virtually all you need in ¼ ounce of whitebait fish, ¼ ounce of cheese, 2 cups of canned sardines, 2 cups of milk, or 1½ ounces of tofu.

magnesium

This is essential for every cell and important to the way calcium and potassium are utilized by your body. You'll find it in cereals, nuts, green vegetables, millet, and whole-wheat bread.

iron

This is vital for blood and the best sources are meat and offal, though whitebait fish, mussels, cockles, and winkles also contain large amounts. Vegetable sources are not so easily absorbed. Get more than your daily dose from 2 ounces of cockles, 5 ounces of liver or 6 ounces of mussels. You can also get valuable amounts of iron from a serving of dahl, a serving of vegetable curry, a serving of beans, or a serving of dark-green vegetables.

potassium

This is needed by every cell but isn't stored by the body. Ensure you get enough by making soups or gravies with the water you've cooked your vegetables in. A large baked potato, a serving of vegetable curry, a dozen dried apricots, a herring or a mackerel, a couple of bananas, a watercress salad, or a handful of raisins, will make up for any deficiencies.

seven-day replenishing

This is a varied week of super-radiant eating during which you'll be making up for all those skin-nourishing and skin- and body-protective nutrients that have not been part of your regular eating in the past.

You can swap whole days around and you can eat light or main meals in whichever order suits your own personal lifestyle, but you must not mix meals from different days.

And during this week, don't drink more than two cups of coffee or black tea a day – that includes decaffeinated versions – but you do need a minimum of one and a half quarts of fluid, one quart of which should be water. The rest can be herb or green tea without milk or sugar.

breakfast rules

Every morning this week you should eat the same breakfast, and there are no excuses for not eating it. It is a major part of your radiance program. If you can find time to get your hair done, fix your make-up, or go to therapy, you can find time for breakfast.

The standard breakfast to be eaten every day consists of:

- A large glass of hot water with a thick slice of unwaxed lemon
- A glass of any fresh unsweetened fruit juice or unsalted vegetable juice
- A portion of any unsweetened whole-grain breakfast cereal, muesli, or hot cereal with soy milk, 4 prunes, and a sprinkling of raisins **or**
- A large glass of soy milk whizzed in a blender with a tablespoon of unsalted shelled nuts, 2 dried apricots, and a banana.

You may also have a cup of tea or coffee.

added extras

Replenishing for Radiance means taking some essential anti-aging skin-, hair- and nail-nourishing nutrients every day. You should stick to this group of supplements for up to six weeks, after which you shouldn't need them unless you have specific health concerns like anemia or menopausal problems, or if you are on long-term medication. In these cases it is beneficial to carry on for longer.

▶ A plant-hormone extract from either soy or red clover
▶ 200 International Units of vitamin E
▶ A one-a-day multi-mineral supplement that includes calcium, potassium, selenium, boron, iodine, and zinc
▶ An anti-oxidant, vitamin, and carotenoid supplement that includes vitamins A, C, E, B6, B12, and folic acid
▶ 500mg evening primrose oil.

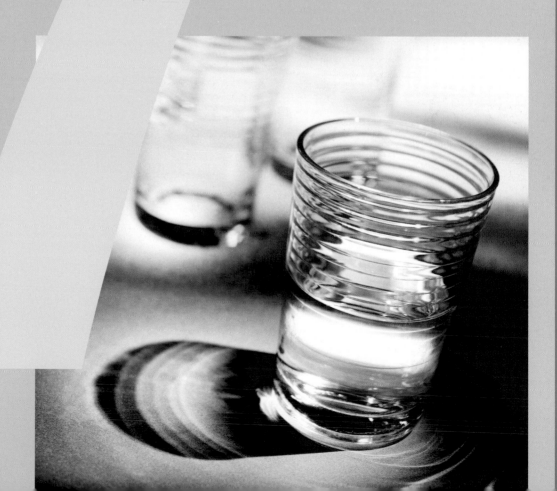

day 1

light meal   Brown Rice Risotto with Sun-Dried Tomatoes (see recipe, page 210) with a salad of chicory, cucumber, carrot, and celery

A thick slice of cantaloupe

main meal   Grilled Sole with Cheese (see recipe, page 215) with steamed broccoli, snow peas, and corn served with olive oil and lemon and sprinkled with toasted pumpkin seeds

A large pear

day 2

light meal   Pasta with Tuna Fish and Black Olives (see recipe, page 218)

A mixed salad with oil-and-vinegar dressing, sprinkled with toasted sunflower seeds

Kiwi and Passion Fruit Smoothie (see recipe, page 191), replacing the milk with soy milk

main meal   Chicken Liver Kebabs (see recipe, page 216) with whole-wheat pita

A large salad of lettuce, arugula, watercress, parsley, and mint with an olive-oil and lemon-juice dressing

Soy, Blueberry, and Strawberry Smoothie (see recipe, page 190)

day 3

light meal   Pita Bread Pizza (see recipe, page 220) with a large bowl of Crudités with Garlic Mayonnaise (see recipe, page 245)

Mixture of dried apricots, dates, and walnuts

main meal   Bean Casserole (see recipe, page 219)

A salad of sliced radishes, green onions, mâche, arugula, and parsley

Spiced Baked Apple (see recipe, page 246)

day 4

light meal   Creamy Mackerel with Eggs (see recipe, page 219) and whole-wheat toast

Sliced avocado and tomato salad sprinkled with toasted sunflower and pumpkin seeds

A fruit salad made from fresh grapefruit and orange with lime juice

main meal   Grilled Paprika Chicken (see recipe, page 221) with new potatoes, pak choi, and green beans sprinkled with chopped garlic and a drizzle of olive oil and lemon juice
Fresh Fruit Brûlée (see recipe, page 250)

day 5

light meal   Pasta with Tuna Fish and Black Olives (see recipe, page 218)
A salad of watercress, beansprouts, chicory, and mushrooms
2 kiwi fruit

main meal   Stir-Fried Turkey Breast with Vegetables and Noodles (see recipe, page 213)
Carrot and Melon Salad (see recipe, page 245)
Spiced Apricots (see recipe, page 248)

day 6

light meal   Chilled Avocado Soup (see recipe, page 234)
Rye crispbread with your favorite cheese
Mango and Soy Milk Smoothie (see recipe, page 191)

main meal   Baked Halibut with Mushrooms (see recipe, page 220) served with brown rice and mixed stir-fried vegetables
Apricot and Almond Crumble (see recipe, page 249)

day 7

light meal   Potato Cakes with Broccoli (see recipe, page 215) with chicory, cucumber, carrot, and celery salad
A small bunch of red grapes

main meal   Chicken with Thyme and Lemon (see recipe, page 220) with boiled rice and Ratatouille (see recipe, page 194)
Stewed Pears with Mascarpone and Cloves (see recipe, page 251)

rebuilding for

Now's the time to think about rebuilding your lifestyle and eating for permanent and easily maintained radiance. Having gotten this far, you really have already made a major impact on your body's ability to protect and maintain all the visible aspects of your radiance – a healthy skin, lustrous hair, and strong, beautiful nails. This is not the time to throw away all these hard-won gains. After all, it hasn't been easy and to follow the plans this far has required a great deal of effort, organization, and self-discipline.

If you follow the Rebuilding for Radiance program, I know from my own patients that most of you will end up incorporating the basic concepts into your everyday life on a permanent basis. Equally important is the fact that if you are also shopping and cooking for a family, the overall health benefits as well as the radiance-boosting effects will be passed on to the others, and particularly to your children, and will become part of their normal eating habits, too.

This rebuilding program should be followed exactly as set out the first time you do it, so that you get a feel for the types of foods that are essential at this stage. However, once you've got the hang of it you will easily work out substitute ingredients and will be able to incorporate favorite recipes that provide the same radiance-boosting benefits, but may fit more comfortably with your own particular likes and dislikes and the lifestyle of you and your family.

The whole object of Rebuilding for Radiance is to provide you with the tools you need to eat an abundance of radiance-boosting foods with the minimum of effort, and in such a way that you hardly have to think about it because it has become a daily routine. Instead of reaching

radiance

for the instant noodles or microwaveable frozen meal, you automatically choose fresh pasta, nuts, and seeds for skin-nourishing minerals, dark green leafy vegetables for their anti-bacterial and skin-protective sulphur compounds, dried fruits for their betacarotene, which is vital for the growth of new skin cells, and soy products for their plant hormones that take care of your hair and skin.

One of the biggest problems I have with my own patients is their sometimes strange and inappropriate concept of what is healthy. Thanks to the lunatic fringe of bogus nutritionists, vast numbers of women have stopped eating a wide range of foods in the belief that they are either fattening or unhealthy, and this includes some of the most important radiance-boosting foods. Something like 30 percent of women believe they're allergic to wheat and dairy products, while in reality less than 2 percent of the population has allergies to these foods. Sadly for these women, both these food groups contain nutrients that hold the key to healthy skin, hair, and nails. Similarly, many women don't eat avocados, one of the richest sources of vitamin E, another essential skin and hair nutrient. A good proportion of women also avoid eggs because of their cholesterol content, but this is yet another of those nutritional myths. Eggs are, in fact, an excellent source of iron, B vitamins, and lecithin – all super-radiance nutrients for skin, hair, and nails.

As I've said before, to rebuild your radiance the simple answer is a diet that combines the widest possible range of different foods. Only this is your guarantee of an optimum intake of radiant nutrients.

fourteen-day rebuilding

This fourteen-day Rebuilding for Radiance regime starts by repeating the seven-day Replenishing for Radiance plan. I'm sure you'll agree that the food was varied and interesting, as well as tasting good. The recipes in it are all extremely healthy and not at all difficult. That makes them perfect for everyone in the family, so you won't need to cook two separate meals all the time.

When it comes to the rebuilding regime, breakfasts loom large again and it really is vital that you eat one of the alternatives every single day. They provide the phytoestrogens that help balance your hormone levels and they are a rich source of B vitamins, fiber, and minerals. On top of that, they give you a combination of instant- and slow-release energy. This is what perks you up in the morning and keeps you going till lunchtime, so you don't have that mid-morning sugar craving that leads to radiance-destroying unhealthy snacks.

During this week do not drink more than four cups of coffee or black tea a day — that includes decaffeinated versions — but you need a minimum of one and a half quarts of fluid, one quart of which should be water. The rest can be herb or green tea without milk or sugar.

You can switch the meals around on each day and even switch whole days, but don't take breakfast from one day, a light meal from another, and a main meal from a third, as this won't give you the daily balance you need.

You should still be taking your Replenishing for Radiance extras and should continue with them throughout this rebuilding regime. Here are your menus for week 2.

Days 1–7, follow the Seven-Day Replenishing program.

day 8

breakfast   A glass of fresh unsweetened fruit juice or unsalted vegetable juice

2 poached eggs and a poached tomato on an unbuttered slice of whole-grain bread (toasted or untoasted)

light meal   Brown Rice Risotto with Sun-Dried Tomatoes (see recipe, page 210) with a salad of chicory, cucumber, carrot, and celery

1 thick slice of Radiance Teabread (see recipe, page 181)

main meal   Salmon Fishcakes with Tomato Salsa (see recipe, page 214) with steamed Chinese cabbage, zucchini, and new potatoes in their skins

Stewed Pears with Mascarpone and Cloves (see recipe, page 251)

day 9

breakfast   A glass of fresh unsweetened fruit juice or unsalted vegetable juice

A large helping of fresh blueberries, raspberries, currants, strawberries – whatever is in season – with a carton of live natural yogurt, sprinkled with 2 teaspoons of wheat germ and 2 teaspoons of toasted linseeds

light meal   Eggplant Caviar with Crudités (see recipe, page 244) with warm whole-wheat pita bread

A fresh fruit salad

main meal   Shrimp and Tomato Curry (see recipe, page 212) with brown rice and mixed green salad

A bowl of live natural yogurt sprinkled with toasted almonds and a drizzle of honey

day 10

breakfast   A glass of fresh unsweetened fruit juice or unsalted vegetable juice

A fresh peach sliced into a bowl of organic low-salt whole-wheat flakes, with chilled soy milk, and 2 teaspoons of flaked almonds

light meal   A sliced avocado with Fava Bean, Tomato, and Herb Salad (see recipe, page 244), with 2 rice cakes

Pink Grapefruit Sorbet (see recipe, page 251)

main meal Corn and Haddock Chowder (see recipe, page 234)

A good chunk of My Easy Bread (see recipe, page 176)

A green leaf salad with fresh chopped mint, thyme, and dill, and a squeeze of lemon juice

A small piece of goat's cheese and a fresh peach

day 11

breakfast A fresh strawberry and banana smoothie made with half live natural yogurt and half soy milk

1 slice of whole-wheat bread or toast with a thin slice of Dutch cheese

light meal A fruit cocktail made from fresh orange, kiwi, and grapefruit

Eggs Florentine (see recipe, page 214) with fingers of whole-wheat toast

Buckwheat Crêpes (see recipe, page 184), sprinkled with raisins and replacing the honey with maple syrup

main meal Spinach Soup with Yogurt (see recipe, page 235)

Quick Chickpea Hot Pot (see recipe, page 215)

A salad of large plum, cherry, and sun-dried tomatoes sprinkled with torn basil and drizzled with olive oil

Any seasonal fresh fruit

day 12

breakfast A glass of fresh unsweetened fruit juice or unsalted vegetable juice

A large bowl of fresh chopped apple, pear, kiwi, mango, and papaya with a generous squeeze of lime juice

1 slice of whole-wheat toast with a little butter and honey

light meal Watercress Soup (see recipe, page 235)

Dark rye bread with a generous portion of your favorite cheeses and an apple and a few grapes

main meal Griddled Tuna with Roasted Vegetables and Fusilli (see recipe, page 222)

Fresh Cherry Tart (see recipe, page 249)

day 13

breakfast A glass of fresh unsweetened fruit juice or unsalted vegetable juice
Colcannon (see recipe, page 180)

light meal A large Greek Salad (see recipe, page 244) with warm whole-wheat pita bread
Yogurt, Papaya, and Kiwi Smoothie (see recipe, page 191)

main meal A salad of baby artichoke hearts, peas, carrots, and mint with olive-oil and cider-vinegar dressing
Chicken Liver Kebabs (see recipe, page 216) on a bed of rice
Any stewed fruit with live yogurt

day 14

breakfast A glass of fresh unsweetened fruit juice or unsalted vegetable juice
Half a pink grapefruit
Cinnamon Toast with Figs (see recipe, page 181)

light meal One-Pot Pasta with Vegetables and Pesto (see recipe, page 223)
Half a honeydew melon filled with mixed berries

main meal Potted Shrimp (see recipe, page 213)
Beef and Ginger Stir-Fry (see recipe, page 224)
A bowl of soaked dried fruits

radiant minds for

Radiance stems from both the physical and the spiritual. You won't have perfect hair, skin, and nails if your body is deficient in essential nutrients or awash with toxic pollutants from food, drink, or the environment. But radiance is multi-factorial and while good nutrition will give you a sound foundation, there are physical and emotional factors that can have a powerful influence – positive or negative – on your radiant state.

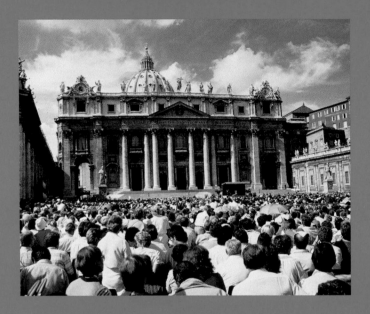

On the emotional side, everyone has to deal with negative emotions such as stress, depression, anger, hate, spite, and jealousy. So that these emotions don't destroy your radiance, you need to learn how to deal with them. Take stress, for example. Not all stress is bad and in fact, you can learn how to use well-controlled stress to your advantage. And when stress does strike, follow my simple tips for keeping it to a minimum (see pages 152–153). You'll see just how well you can survive and keep your radiance intact.

On the physical side, age-old therapies such as massage and aromatherapy can give a huge boost to your overall feelings of well-being, and these will complement the nutritional radiance benefits gained from your already improved diet. Part of the radiance benefits of massage come from the healing power of touch, regardless of the type of massage, but the benefits

radiant bodies

don't come only from a professional massage. In fact, there's no reason why anyone shouldn't give a massage to a friend or partner as, with very few exceptions, it's impossible to do any harm. And perhaps the most surprising fact is that the giver derives almost as much radiance-boosting benefit as the receiver. I know. I've been doing it for 40 years. Just try for yourself.

Another facet to the physical side of radiance is activity. Few people make this association, but without a shadow of doubt, regular exercise benefits your overall well-being, your heart and circulation, and consequently your skin and hair. In terms of your overall well-being, it generates the release of the brain's own feel-good chemicals – endorphins – so after exercise you won't just glow from exertion, but also from happy, radiant feelings. Physical activity will also increase the amount of oxygen in your blood and will stimulate your heart rate and the amount of blood pumped through your system. This in turn will carry more nutrients to your skin and hair follicles, and the result will be healthier and more radiant skin and hair. But whatever you do, don't be tempted to become a marathon runner or an obsessive exerciser as doing this will have a serious negative impact on your radiance and general health. Modest exercise three or four times a week is all you need.

And last but not least comes radiance-boosting laughter. Although you may think it sounds like an old wives' tale, laughter really is the best medicine, and there's now a lot of scientific evidence to prove it. But you don't need me to tell you that – watching somebody who is smiling and laughing is a much more radiant vision than sitting opposite someone at dinner whose mouth is permanently turned down and whose brow is furrowed in a frown.

beat the stress

Some stress is essential to normal life and it's often the adrenaline generated by stress that powers creativity. The problems occur when stress becomes relentless and excessive. Apart from the repercussions on your health – high blood pressure, strokes, heart disease, anxiety, insomnia, and a host of other medical problems – nothing affects your radiance to the same degree. Your posture suffers and you droop. The blood supply to your skin is diminished, and you look gray and puffy. Constant tension and anxiety lead to headaches, which result in frowning and worry lines. None of this makes you feel or look your radiant best.

You may not realize how much stress you're under, so how do you tell whether you are suffering from too much? Check the questionnaire below and see how you score. Do you:

▶ feel near to tears much of the time?
▶ fidget, bite your nails, or fiddle with your hair?
▶ find it hard to concentrate and impossible to make decisions?
▶ find it increasingly hard to talk to people?
▶ snap and shout at those around you at home and work?
▶ eat when you're not hungry?
▶ feel tired much of the time?
▶ think that your sense of humor has gone for good?
▶ feel suspicious of others?
▶ no longer have any interest in sex?
▶ sleep badly?
▶ drink and/or smoke more to help you through those difficult days?
▶ ever feel that you just can't cope?

If you answer **yes** to more than four of these questions, you are stressed. **Do something!** You can't carry on this way.

de-stress the distress

Here's how to break out of the cycle.

▶ Do not work more than nine hours a day.

▶ Take at least half an hour off in the day.

▶ Take at least one and a half days out of your normal working routine each week.

▶ Eat regular and healthy meals.

▶ Take regular exercise.

▶ Practice some form of relaxation technique.

▶ Do not use alcohol, caffeine, nicotine, or drugs to relieve stress.

▶ Remember that stressful situations are not always the unhappy ones. Getting married, promoted, or moving all cause stress.

▶ Learn to recognize your own stress thresholds.

▶ Use stress positively and channel your energy into making your life better.

get rid of your anger

Just like excessive stress, anger causes resentment, bitterness, and anxiety. If you let it get the better of you, it not only damages your health, but has a powerful negative effect on how radiant you look and feel. Not surprisingly, the trick is to learn to let your anger out.

Attitudes to letting go of your anger vary enormously in different parts of the world. For example, the Anglo-Saxon approach is very different from the Mediterranean one. If you're Anglo-Saxon, it's not acceptable to lose your temper, but watch an Italian, Spanish, or Greek family eating Sunday lunch and from all the shouting and gesticulating, you'd imagine they were in the middle of a 50-year feud. In reality, they're probably only arguing about whether there's too much salt in the soup.

People from the Mediterranean have no inhibitions about showing their anger and I'm sure this is why in the Mediterranean, even great-grandmothers, weather-beaten and wrinkled though they may be, exude boundless radiance.

how to let go

There are many ways to release the pent-up anger and frustrations of day-to-day living, and it's far safer to do so in a controlled and purposeful way than to let the pressure build and build until you finally get sick or explode into a violent rage.

Physical exercise is especially recommended by the experts. It gets rid of excess energy, encourages self-confidence, and offers a safe environment for you to use your anger in a competitive way. It's known, for example, that endurance runners, who run long distances each week, tend to be less anxious, more emotionally stable, and less prone to irrational outbursts of anger than their physically less active contemporaries.

If sport's not your thing, find out what works for you. For some, it's a hobby like gardening or painting; for others, movies, theater, or music.

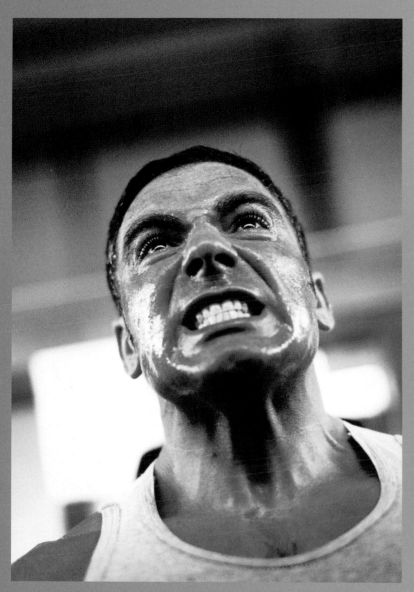

I was once at the Tivoli Gardens in Copenhagen where the local pottery had a stand full of their seconds. For just a small cost, you could hurl a pile of reject plates at a brick wall. It was a perfect way to get rid of any anger. If you don't happen to have a handy store of old china, try hanging a rug in the garden and beating it with a tennis racket, or having a punching bag in your bedroom. Then, after a frustrating day when the boss has been on your back or you've been given a parking ticket, you can have a five-minute workout. Hit and punch away, shout and scream, just lose your inhibitions. You'll be amazed at how relaxed and calm you feel afterward. It's all too easy to criticize people who have a short fuse, but unless their anger turns to violence, they are better off than people who, as a result of years of conditioning, find it impossible to show any anger or annoyance.

If you're in any doubt, just think of the fun you had last time you smashed some plates at a Greek taverna!

smile and the world smiles with you

To boost your radiance even more, you must remember to smile. It requires much more effort to frown than to smile, as frowning uses many more muscles. And it's frowning that leaves you with a wrinkled forehead, droopy skin at the corners of your eyes, and a miserable down-turned mouth. Smiling on the other hand makes you feel good and look radiant. And surprising though it may seem, smiling brings skin-protective benefits. There's now a mass of scientific evidence proving conclusively that positive attitudes enhance the body's immune defenses and so protect your skin – and all your other organs too – from the aging damage of free radicals.

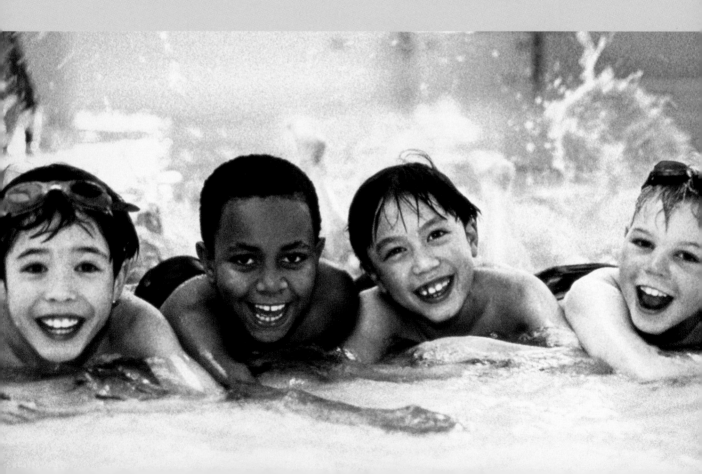

rude noises can be good for your face

As a result of watching children playing games with straws and drinks, I developed a range of exercises which I have used on my patients for many years to help them recover facial muscle strength after strokes and other neurological problems. Over the years I've seen that these simple exercises have cosmetic benefits, too. They build excellent tone in your facial muscles, which in turn support the structure of your skin. They also stimulate the blood flow to the cells of the skin and the skin's nerve supply. Making this small effort will repay you with a very large radiance dividend, so I strongly recommend these as a regular part of your ongoing radiance therapy. Repeat each exercise three times and try and repeat all ten at least three times a week. Do them in front of you partner, children, or grandchildren and everyone will have a good laugh as well – and as you know, laughter is the best medicine.

All you need are a large glass of water and a package of thick plastic straws.

1 With the straw in the middle of your lips and the other end under the water, breathe in through your nose and very slowly out through the straw to produce a constant stream of bubbles.

2 Repeat as above, but with the straw in the left-hand corner of your mouth.

3 Repeat as above, but in the right hand-corner of your mouth.

4 Suck a mouthful of water through the straw as quickly as you can and swallow.

5 Suck a mouthful of water as slowly as you can and swallow.

6 Suck a mouthful of water and blow it back into the glass as quickly as you can.

7 Suck a mouthful of water and blow it back into the glass as slowly as you can.

8 Blow air through the straw into the water as hard as you can with your cheeks held in.

9 Blow air through the straw into the water as hard as you can with your cheeks puffed out.

10 Do this exercise in front of a mirror – raise your left eyebrow, raise your right eyebrow, purse your lips, blow a raspberry, suck in your cheeks, blow out your cheeks, blow another raspberry.

simple extras for added radiance

Throughout history, foods have been used both internally and externally for the treatment of virtually every ailment. Enhancing radiance is no exception and for many simple radiance-boosting applications you need look no further than your own kitchen.

There are really considerable advantages when you make your own kitchen remedies to use on your skin, hands, nails, and hair. First, they are incredibly cheap. Second, you avoid the damaging chemical additives that are used in the vast majority of commercially available products, but third, and most important, these kitchen remedies work better than most things that you buy over the counter from the pharmacy or the beauty shop – and you're not paying for all the excessive advertising or the environmentally damaging packaging.

Many of these do-it-yourself radiance products are simplicity itself– a pitcher of camomile tea as a hair rinse, a bowl of warm olive oil to nourish the fingernails, garlic and vinegar to cure fungal infections, rosewater and glycerin for beautiful smooth hands, lemon juice to clean and whiten cuticles. You'll find how to use oats as one of the simplest of radiance-boosting skin nourishers and if you like chocolate, you'll discover a new use for it in this section of the book. There are even enzymes in pineapple that are good for your hands. And when it comes to hair the choice is endless. Apart from natural plant colorings, you can use artichoke, catmint, witch hazel, or tea tree oil as a dandruff treatment, and you can even make your own shampoos for oily or dry hair.

Although hair and nails are extremely important when it comes to your total radiant look, it's the skin which most women worry about and this is where kitchen medicine really comes into its own. Cider vinegar, almonds, eggs, tomatoes, and live yogurt, as well as fruits such as mangoes, peaches, and avocados, and vegetables like cucumbers and cabbage, can all be made up into external applications for a wide variety of skin problems, ranging from dry skin, oily skin, pimples, and blemishes to acne, eczema, and psoriasis. But this is just the tip of the iceberg. You can also use essential oils and fresh herbs to make steam infusions or to add to your bath, there are special honeys to treat infections, and the most effective remedy of all for boils is still the old-fashioned bread poultice which has been in regular use for at least 300 years.

I urge you to try these really simple radiance treats. They're fun to make, using them will give you the greatest of pleasure, and you'll find that they really do work.

When it comes to supplements and extras to boost your radiance, I mostly recommend those that are based on natural products that have an inherent anti-inflammatory effect or that are rich in the plant hormones (phytoestrogens). These play a vital role in regulating hormonal balance, which is of particular importance for women who have irregular periods, suffer with Premenstrual Syndrome (PMS), or who are just beginning or have had menopause. They are even more essential for women who have had a premature menopause, whether due to surgery, illness, anorexia, or any other reason, as they may be the key to increased protection against osteoporosis, skin aging, and early heart disease.

kitchen remedies for skin

As we've already seen, eating lots of processed, packaged, and convenience foods is certain to have an adverse effect on your skin, and alcohol and caffeine wreak havoc, too. Obviously, the first thing to do is detox and improve your diet long term, but meanwhile there are also some wonderful skin treatments you can produce in your very own kitchen.

live yogurt and salt scrub

This is one of the simplest kitchen remedies for skin. Simply add 2 teaspoons of coarse sea salt to a carton of yogurt, spread it evenly all over your face and leave for 10 minutes. Then, using cold water, gently rub the mixture all over the skin until it's rinsed off completely. The salt acts as a gentle exfoliator and antiseptic and the natural bacteria in the yogurt provide a protective layer that will fight off any other bugs and help to prevent the formation of pimples. It's worth doing this at least twice a week.

oats

These are a wonderful emollient for any inflamed skin. Put 4 tablespoons of uncooked oats in a muslin bag, hang the bag under the taps as you run the bath, then use the bag to clean your skin. The natural oils and vitamins in the oats will soothe inflamed areas and stimulate the growth of new skin. Use for three or four baths before replacing the oats.

avocados

These are nature's gift to the skin. They are not only wonderfully nutritious, but avocado oil makes a great skin food. After you've eaten your avocado, rub your skin with the inside of the peel and massage in the oily film that's left behind.

comfrey, calendula (from the marigold plant), and camomile

These are three herbs that can easily be grown in your own garden and have unique powers to soften, soothe, protect, and heal the skin. Comfrey promotes the growth or regeneration of skin tissue; calendula clears up any infection – fungal, viral, or bacterial – and counters inflammation; and camomile soothes, heals, and stimulates cell regeneration. Make up a strong infusion of all three, cool and strain it, then use it as a facial rinse or added to your bath.

oranges

These make a delicious face mask. Purée the pulp of a whole orange, spread it over your face, leave for 20 minutes, then rinse off with tepid water. This leaves the skin feeling clean and stimulated. Your skin will also have absorbed some of the orange's vitamin C, betacarotene, and a complex of bioflavonoids called vitamin P which strengthen the tiny capillaries, so protecting you from unsightly broken veins.

Face masks are also good made from honey, carrot grated into olive oil, and grape juice (or peeled and crushed fresh grapes).

lavender

This has been known for years to do wonders for the skin. Steep the tops of fresh lavender sprigs in white wine vinegar for a week (shake the bottle occasionally), then dilute 1 part of the vinegar to 4 parts of water and use as a skin tonic.

almond oil

This is used as a base for many natural skin products. You can make your own oil treatments by adding a couple of drops of your favorite essential oil to a tablespoon of almond oil. For oily skin, use chamomile, lavender, or rose, while neroli or clary sage are good for older skins. Spread the oil mixture on your face and leave for 20 minutes before washing off and applying a skin tonic.

fresh herbs

These are great for a facial sauna. Put a handful into a pan, pour boiling water over, cover the pan, leave to infuse for 10 minutes, then reheat. Remove from the heat, transfer to a heatproof bowl and lean over the steaming bowl with a towel over your head. Choose from lavender to heal and soothe the skin, rosemary to heal and stimulate the circulation, marigold to heal and cornflower to refresh. Mallow, marigold, and sage are particularly good for problem skins, comfrey and borage flowers are great for dry skin, and thyme will open your pores and get your blood really pumping.

kitchen remedies for hair

When your hair is looking less than radiant, it's often an early warning sign that you're not well. Your hairdresser will often notice a deterioration in the condition of your hair or scalp before any other symptoms appear. Once you've detoxed, you'll be well on the way to regaining a lovely head of hair, but some simple kitchen remedies can help too. And this isn't just for the ladies. Although men are much more likely to lose their hair, that's no excuse for not taking the best possible care of it while you can.

jojoba oil

This conditions and adds luster to the hair. Heat a couple of tablespoons of jojoba oil, apply it to the roots, then comb it through the hair. Wrap a warm towel around your head and leave it for 30 minutes, then use a very mild shampoo to wash out the oil.

ginger root with sesame oil

Together these make a very stimulating conditioner. Squeeze the juice of the fresh root into a couple of tablespoons of oil, apply to the hair and wrap your head in a warm towel. Leave it on for as long as possible before shampooing.

rosemary

Traditionally used to stimulate local blood circulation. Add a handful to cold water, simmer for 15 minutes, then swab the roots of your hair with the mixture before shampooing.

nettles

Nettles are rich in the minerals needed for healthy growth. Try to wash your hair daily in a mild non-detergent nettle shampoo. Steam young nettletops to eat with a knob of butter and a little nutmeg, then use the steaming water to rub into your scalp.

onion

This is a wonderful source of sulphur, which is essential for healthy hair. As well as including onions in your diet, rubbing raw onion over the roots of your hair before you shampoo will stimulate your scalp.

for dandruff

Use a camomile shampoo, and add a cup of cider vinegar to 2 cups of hot water for the final rinse. In addition, massage your scalp thoroughly at bedtime with witch hazel extract or add a few drops of tea tree oil to your normal shampoo. You can also make a final rinse from a dozen or so globe artichoke leaves, simmered for 10 minutes, strained and cooled, or from catmint tea – a generous handful of chopped catmint leaves steeped in boiling water for 10 minutes, strained, and left to cool.

for fair hair

To enhance blond hair, make a final rinse from an infusion of mullein, strained and cooled, or from camomile or from nettle teabag.

for dark hair

Condition with a solution of 1 cup of beet juice to 4 cups of hot water with a teaspoon of salt. Massage through the hair, then rinse out.

to cover gray

Avoid horrible commercial dyes yet cover your gray by using sage. Add 4 large spoons of chopped leaves to a pitcher of boiling water, cover, and leave for at least half an hour before straining. Use a brush or sponge to apply the liquid to the gray roots. Don't wash out.

for dry hair and flaky scalp

Warm a cup of olive oil in a bowl of hot water, massage it into the scalp and hair, wrap your head in a towel for 1 hour, then shampoo, and rinse with the camomile and cider-vinegar mix (see above).

For dry hair on its own, add an egg yolk and a teaspoon of natural gelatin dissolved in a little boiling water to your favorite herbal shampoo.

for oily hair

To make the ideal shampoo for oily hair, mix together half a cup of rosewater, 2 whole eggs and a generous dash of dark rum.

kitchen remedies for nails and hands

You can be perfectly groomed from head to toe, but roughened skin on your hands and cracked, flaking, ridged, or fungus-infected nails are impossible to hide. They can't help but detract from the radiant impression the rest of you is making. But never fear. Help is at hand as kitchen remedies once again come to your radiance rescue.

fungal nail infections

These are a common problem and very unsightly, but are easy to treat yourself. Eat plenty of garlic for its powerful anti-fungal properties, but also bathe the affected nails in a mixture of 1 cup of warm water, 1 tablespoon of cider vinegar and 2 pressed or minced cloves of garlic. This will help athlete's foot as well.

brittle nails

Make sure you eat 2 teaspoons of extra-virgin olive oil each day and once a week soak your nails in a bowl of warm olive oil. After 10 minutes, wipe off the surplus. You can also strengthen your nails by soaking them in an infusion of dried horsetail.

reddened or chafed hands

Almonds and almond oil are kind to chafed hands. Make a soft paste of ground almonds and a little rosewater and spread it on your hands like a face mask. Leave on for about half an hour, then wipe off the surplus. Alternatively, mix together equal parts of rosewater and glycerin and rub into your hands at bedtime. You can wear soft cotton gloves during the night to boost the effect.

Essential oils also help rough hands. In a small bottle, mix $3^{1}/_{2}$ tablespoons of almond oil with 25 drops of camomile, lavender, or benzoin, and add a vitamin E capsule. Warm the bottle under hot tap water, then at bedtime just massage the mixture in and sleep tight. To prevent your hands getting rough in the first place, use a barrier cream for harsh or dirty jobs. In my opinion, the best is this one that you can make at home. Mix together $1/8$ ounce of kaolin (stocked by most pharmacies), $1/8$ ounce of cold-pressed almond oil, and the yolk of a large organic egg. Rub the mixture well into your hands, particularly around the cuticles and under the nails and when you've finished your dirty tasks, simply scrub off with a soft bristle brush, leaving your hands clean and the skin soft and undamaged.

lemons

Always have fresh lemons in your kitchen. The flesh and juice rubbed into your hands not only help keep your hands clean but they whiten the skin, are strongly antiseptic, and are an effective deodorant if you've been handling onions, garlic, or fish.

oats

There's now a large range of oat-based commercial products for hand and skin care on the market, but save your money. Simply take a scoop of oats out of your package, put them in your cupped hand, add some water and rub your hands together until the oats form a paste. Massage this thoroughly in every nook and cranny of your hands, fingers, cuticles, and nails, then rinse off. The fiber is an effective cleanser, but you also absorb vitamin E and other radiance-boosting nutrients through the skin.

chocolate

Sorry, you don't get to eat it! But if you've had a heavy session in the garden, been redecorating the house, or your job involves working with tools so you end up with calloused, hard hands, mix cocoa butter, beeswax, and cold-pressed almond oil in equal proportions and heat them very slowly in a heatproof bowl over a saucepan of boiling water. When they've all dissolved together, remove from the heat and keep stirring until the mixture sets. Keep in a jam jar wrapped in foil and use as hand cream every night.

pineapple

Fresh pineapple contains the enzyme bromelaine which is a highly effective digestive enzyme that also softens the cuticles. Make a large glass of fresh pineapple juice, put 2 tablespoons into a jug with 1 scant teaspoon of cider vinegar and 1 teaspoon of extra-virgin olive oil. Whisk together and soak your nails for at least 15 minutes. Drink the rest of the juice!

supplements and natural remedies for lifelong radiance

I've already said it, but I'll say it again – no supplements are a substitute for healthy eating. But when it comes to radiance, there are a number of supplements and natural remedies that can provide a real boost. These are not "magic bullets." Think of them rather as insurance that will give you the best possible chance of radiant good health when you're young, of feeling and looking great in your middle years, and of basking in that quiet glow of radiant energy, beautiful skin, and healthy hair and nails which is especially important to our sense of self-esteem and well-being when we are older.

natural plant hormones

The natural plant hormones that can be extracted from soy beans, red clover, and other plant material can be of major benefit in terms of maintaining and protecting your natural radiance. These are all available as supplements and, as with virtually all medicines, finding the one that suits you best is a simple question of trial and error. They are particularly important in the treatment of acne, skin problems related to irregular periods, hormone imbalance, polycystic ovarian syndrome, adult acne, and at all stages of women's menopausal years – pre-, during and post-menopause.

essential fatty acids

These crop up time and time again as natural anti-inflammatories, for dealing with skin problems and for women's health problems in general, but there is now such an overwhelming body of scientific evidence that demonstrates their need that they can't be ignored as a radiance protector and booster as well as for their more medicinal benefits.

Under this umbrella come the hugely beneficial cod-liver oil, fish oil, evening primrose oil, canola oil, and flax-seed oil. I'm afraid that the bad news for vegetarians and vegans is that there really is no substitute for the fish oils and though I know that most vegetarians and vegans would never eat oily fish, I really do urge them to take a supplement, especially if they're planning pregnancy or are pregnant or breastfeeding – if not for their own sake, then for that of their baby.

herbs and spices

Tried and tested through the years as radiance boosters, many herbs and spices are easy to grow or readily available in your supermarket, health food shop, or greengrocer.

parsley

This is a gentle diuretic which helps the body get rid of fluid. It's also rich in vitamins A and C, and is a reasonable source of iron. Make it into Parsley Tea (see recipe, page 189) and drink a glass every day. You'll find it's wonderful for the skin.

thyme

One of the most powerful anti-viral and anti-bacterial herbs, it protects against all forms of infection, particularly skin and stomach bugs. Add to tomato, cheese, egg, or salad recipes.

cloves

A great aid to digestion and a help in the treatment of irritable bowel syndrome. Anything that improves digestive output means better skin and clearer eyes. Use it when cooking fruits and in stews and casseroles made from lamb, game, or venison.

basil

A superb remedy for tension and anxiety headaches – a common cause of frowning and wrinkles – but it also has a gentle calming and soothing action which will help you relax and unwind. It's also useful in improving irregular periods.

sage

This is particularly important as we get older, as sage helps to improve short-term memory and is also a strong protector against infections. For women approaching menopause, sage helps even out hormone imbalances and reduces the risk of sudden aging of the skin, breaking nails, hair loss, and hot flashes. Use lots of it in cooking and drink a cup of sage tea daily – a teaspoon of chopped sage leaves to a cup of boiling water.

posture and color for radiant looks

Stop and think for a moment about the last time you couldn't help but stare at someone in the street, getting out of a car, or standing next to you at the supermarket checkout. You were no doubt wondering what made that person look so special. Regardless of age, sex, or wealth, there are people whose radiance just shouts above the crowd. It's that indefinable combination of the way they move, their wonderful posture and deportment based on strong bones, and their innate sense of color.

Few people make the link between radiance and posture but it is very real. We're all born with good posture. You only have to look at the way babies hold themselves when they first start to sit, crawl, and walk. Their bodies achieve good posture naturally and with the minimum amount of effort. Unfortunately, though, learned behavior soon takes over and thanks to badly designed furniture, acquired habits, sitting all day at a computer, lack of exercise, and general laziness, our bodies suffer from chronic misalignment and we need a much greater muscular effort to hold ourselves up. This results in muscular tension and physical problems like head, neck, shoulder, and low back pain. Often we have breathing and digestive difficulties, too. Every movement we make drains our energy resources.

None of this contributes to our radiance. But for contrast, just think about those wonderful African and Asian women carrying bundles on their heads who seem to glide across the ground with such effortless grace. As you will see on the following pages, a combination of yoga, Alexander Technique, and simple weight-bearing exercises can help you overcome your bad habits and relearn the art of graceful posture and movement.

The next step is to learn about the power of color to unleash the new, radiant you. It's easy to scoff at the concept of color therapy and to believe that it's a holdover from the hippy Sixties or just the latest bit of twenty-first century psychobabble, but nothing could be further from the truth. Color has been used as a mood-enhancing and therapeutic tool for at least two thousand years. Shamans, mystics, the physicians of ancient Greece, and psychiatrists – all have discovered the immense power of color.

Today, industrial psychologists advise companies on the best colors to use in offices, factories, and workshops in order to enhance the work people do on these premises. And in the past, people who could afford it painted the rooms of their house in different colors according to the activities that went on there – reds for dining rooms to stimulate conversation and the intellect, greens for the library to aid concentration and calm when reading, the palest yellows for the most restful bedrooms, and terracotta and pinks for elegant, restrained sitting rooms.

Now we know that it's what you wear that matters, too. As I'll show you, you can learn to dress for the occasion, so the colors you wear enhance the mood you need to feel and convey – whether it's for that special business meeting, for that interview for a new job, for a blind date, or for a romantic dinner for two.

improve your posture

If you're trying to unlock your radiance, the key isn't simply to slap on more make-up in an attempt to cover up the flaws. Instead, you need to concentrate on improving your mobility, flexibility, and bone strength. Fortunately, there are many tried and tested ways of doing this, ranging from yoga and Alexander technique to simple weight-bearing exercises that help keep the dreaded osteoporosis at bay.

yoga

Yoga is great for inner and outer radiance. It is a profoundly religious and spiritual system that has existed in India for thousands of years. In the West, it is mostly associated with a range of distinctive postures that promote mobility and flexibility and that also have therapeutic benefits for many parts of the body. Combining the postures with traditional yoga breathing helps establish patterns of profound relaxation and inner peace which can combat the lunatic pace of life that most of us live at in the twenty-first century.

Yoga is ideal for people of any age. You can learn the simple poses from books and videos but it's always best to learn from an experienced teacher, who will ensure that you achieve the positions with the minimum effort and without risk of injury. For maximum benefit, once you're familiar with the postures, you need to practice on a daily basis.

alexander technique

Alexander was a struggling actor who discovered that his voice problems were caused by tension and bad posture. He developed his system to deal with these and over the years it has become hugely popular with dancers, musicians, and performers of all kinds.

It offers a process of physical re-education that has far-reaching effects. For example, it can help with many conditions such as asthma, migraine, high blood pressure, backache, and bowel problems. As far as your radiance is concerned, it will also help you move better so you look better, but even more importantly, it has a positive effect on your circulation and breathing. This will improve the oxygen-carrying ability of your blood, which means more nutrients will be delivered to your skin.

Alexander is one technique that you cannot learn from books, videos, or the Internet. Alexander practitioners think of themselves as teachers and their clients as pupils, and their job is to re-educate the postural bad habits that you've developed during your life. An Alexander teacher will gently realign your body to re-establish the perfect relationship between your head, neck, and trunk. The technique also focuses on discovering how to use the minimum muscular effort required to achieve any single task. Through constant practice and learning to become aware of what you are doing, you will gradually come to feel uncomfortable with your bad old postural habits and will recognize what feels good and healthy.

weight-bearing exercise

One in three women and one in twelve men will develop osteoporosis and tragically it's happening in younger and younger people. Apart from eating a diet rich in calcium and vitamin D, the major protective factor against this life-destroying and aging disease is weight-bearing exercise. Although most bone-building goes on during the late teens, it's never too late to encourage your bones to strengthen themselves. You can get your exercise in any way that you enjoy, but you have to have your weight on your feet, so swimming and cycling don't count. A brisk 20-minute walk four times a week is all you need.

boost your radiance with color

Do you automatically wear black, gray, or beige clothes? Many of you will answer "yes" and your excuse will be, "because they're fashionable at the moment." But did you know that colors like these that make you "invisible" can also feed negative emotions such as sadness and depression? And once you're feeling down, you'll inevitably choose these colors, which means you're trapped in a downward spiral – none of which does your radiance any favors. But don't despair. There is a way out. Once you know a few tricks, you can use color to your advantage in many situations – and give your radiance a boost at the same time.

Many color therapy practitioners draw on elements of the ancient Indian art of Ayurvedic medicine and combine it with modern, scientific evidence. In Ayurvedic medicine, light and color are regarded as two of the fundamental life forces which link the body's energy lines, or chakras. These, in turn, govern both our physical and our emotional state. Scientific evidence more or less supports this idea, suggesting that the whole spectrum of colors and wavelengths can have a profound effect on our mental and physical state.

As a general principle, scientific research tells us that red and yellow are the most strongly stimulating colors, while black and blue are the most calming. Many experiments have shown how changing a color scheme can, for example, improve or reduce office productivity, performance on the factory floor, children's learning ability, and people's physical and intellectual skills in a variety of situations.

A number of color therapists also believe that every wavelength has its own vibrational frequency, which adds potency to the mix, but there's no scientific evidence to support this theory. Nevertheless, it's my experience that it doesn't matter whether you can see the colors you're wearing, the mere fact that you are wearing them is enough to change your mood – so perhaps it's the vibrations playing their part.

try it yourself

If you have to abide by a dress code at work, then add some splashes of color. For example, if you're going to a meeting that you know will be stressful, women can try wearing a pale blue scarf or men a pale blue pocket handkerchief. This calming and soothing color will help keep both you and your colleagues' stress levels down.

For complex financial negotiations, when you know you'll need to concentrate hard, add some yellow – men can wear yellow braces, women yellow shoes or a yellow handbag. And if you know you're in for a very long and boring conference program, then we're back to red. This stimulating color will help keep you and those around you awake, and you'll still be looking good at the end of the day.

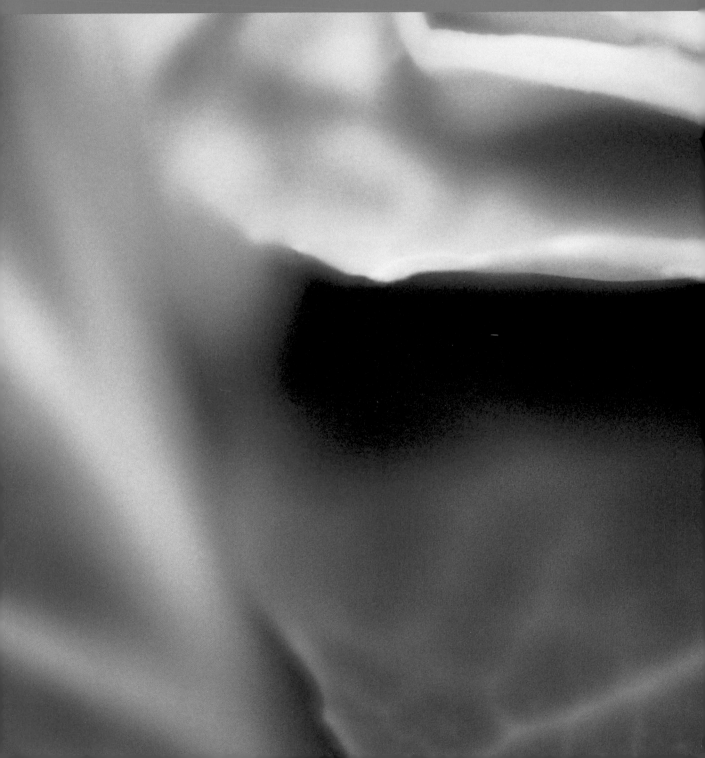

part 4

super detox recipes

all recipes serve 4, except drinks recipes which serve 2

bread and breakfast

my easy bread

stone-ground organic whole-wheat bread flour	4½ cups
fast-rising yeast	1 envelope
extra-virgin olive oil	2 tsp, plus extra for oiling
molasses, dark dark brown sugar or honey	1 tsp
salt	½ tsp
warm water	2 cups
sunflower seeds (optional)	2 tbsp

Good bread is a vital part of any healthy diet, but most commercial bread contains added chemicals that you don't want, as well as far too much salt, which causes fluid retention and reduces the body's natural cleansing and detoxing abilities. The answer is to make your own.

Lightly oil a 1kg loaf pan and keep it warm. Mix the flour and yeast together in a large bowl. Dissolve the olive oil, molasses, sugar or honey and salt in the water. Make a well in the center of the flour and pour in the warm water mixture and sunflower seeds, if using.

Mix all the ingredients together with a wooden spoon, then knead for about 4 minutes, until the dough forms a ball. Put it into the warm pan, cover with a damp dish towel and leave to rise in a warm place for about 40 minutes or until it has risen almost to the top of the pan. Meanwhile, preheat the oven to 400°F.

Transfer the pan to the preheated oven and bake for about 40 minutes, until it sounds hollow when you tap the bottom of the pan. When it's ready, remove from the oven and when it's cool enough to handle, transfer to a wire rack to cool completely.

porridge muesli

uncooked oats	8 heaped tbsp
raisins	4 heaped tsp
apples	2, large
lemon	juice of ½
light cream	4 tbsp

Put the oats into a bowl. Add the raisins and about 6 tbsp of cold water. Cover with plastic wrap and leave overnight. Before serving in the morning, grate the apples into the bowl, add the lemon juice and stir in the cream.

poached eggs and tomatoes

cider or white wine vinegar	1 tsp
tomatoes	4
eggs	4
whole-wheat bread	4 slices
butter	for spreading

Fill a large, deep-sided frying pan with water. Add the vinegar – it helps prevent the egg whites from "fraying." Add the whole tomatoes to the pan, bring to the boil and reduce to a simmer. Roll the eggs, in their shells, in the water for about 15 seconds – again to keep the whites intact. Break the eggs into the water and continue simmering for about 4 minutes. Meanwhile, toast the bread and butter it. Using a slotted spoon, remove the eggs from the water and place on the toast. Remove the tomatoes with a slotted spoon, rub off their skins and serve with the eggs and toast.

fresh fruit kebabs

Simple, impressive, and wonderfully healthy as part of your detox regime.

wooden skewers	4
pineapple	1, small, peeled and cubed
seedless blue or purple grapes	about 1 cup, large
apple	1, cored and cubed
pears	2, cored and cubed
honey	4 tbsp
ground cloves	4 pinches

Soak the skewers in water for 30 minutes before using to prevent burning. Preheat the broiler to high and line the broiler pan with foil. Make sure the pieces of fruit are roughly the same size and thread them on to the skewers. Put the kebabs on the foil-lined broiler pan, drizzle with the honey and sprinkle with the ground cloves. Broil for 2 minutes, then serve.

dutch breakfast

Being half Dutch, I grew up sharing this typical breakfast with my father. It's worth getting a cheese slicer, though you can buy packs of sliced good Dutch cheese. Cheese contains health-giving calcium, protein, vitamin C and fiber and this recipe is very quick to make.

whole-wheat bread	4 slices
butter	for spreading
Gouda cheese	4 thin slices
tomatoes	4, thinly sliced

Simplicity itself . . . just toast the bread and spread with the butter. Top with the cheese slices, then the tomatoes and serve.

poached haddock with cherry tomatoes

Haddock is a wonderful source of protein and minerals, particularly iodine, which controls the thyroid gland – the key to effective detoxing as it stimulates the metabolism.

whole or 2 percent milk	about 1½ cups
butter	4 tbsp
undyed smoked haddock fillets	4, weighing about 6 ounces each
cherry tomatoes	12
black pepper	to taste
parsley	4 large sprigs

Fill a large, deep-sided frying pan with the milk. Add the butter and bring to the boil. Place the fish in the pan and simmer for 5–7 minutes, depending on the thickness of the fish. Add the cherry tomatoes 1 minute before the end of the cooking time to warm through. Drain the fish and tomatoes and transfer to a serving plate. Season with generous grindings of coarsely ground black pepper and garnish with the parsley.

kedgeree

brown, long-grain rice	⅔ cup
cod or undyed smoked haddock	4 ounces
2 percent milk	enough to poach the fish
eggs	2
shrimp (optional)	8, large, cooked and peeled
curry powder	1 tsp
parsley	1 tbsp finely chopped leaves
lemon	juice of ½
butter	2tbsp

Rinse the rice and cook according to the package instructions. Meanwhile, put the fish into a large, deep-sided frying pan, add enough milk to cover and bring slowly to the boil. As soon as it begins to boil, remove from the heat. Cover and let stand for 10 minutes. Remove the fish from the pan with a slotted spoon, then skin and flake it, removing all the bones. While the rice is cooking, poach the eggs.

Drain the rice thoroughly and fluff up with a fork. While it's still warm, gently stir in the shrimp, flaked fish, curry powder, most of the parsley, lemon juice, and butter. Transfer the rice mixture to serving plates, arrange a poached egg on top and sprinkle with the remaining parsley. Serve immediately.

tomato and mushroom omelette

butter	6 tbsp
tomatoes	8, roughly chopped
button mushrooms	4 ounces, wiped and roughly chopped
eggs	10
basil	4 heaped tbsp roughly torn leaves

Melt the butter in a large omelette or nonstick frying pan. Add the tomatoes and mushrooms, cover, and simmer gently for 10 minutes. Remove the vegetables with a slotted spoon and reserve until required. Beat the eggs, pour a quarter of the mixture into the pan, drawing the mixture in from the sides and tilting the pan to make sure you have an even layer. As soon as the omelette begins to set, add a quarter of the tomato and mushroom mixture and swirl around to make sure it is evenly distributed. Cook for 1–2 minutes to brown underneath. Slide the omelette onto a serving plate and sprinkle with a quarter of the basil leaves. Repeat to make the other 3 omelettes.

zucchini and Cheddar omelette

butter	2 tbsp
eggs	8, large
zucchini	2, grated
Cheddar cheese	½ cup, grated
cucumber	¼, peeled and finely sliced

Melt the butter in a large omelette or nonstick frying pan over a low heat. Beat 4 of the eggs and add to the pan. As soon as the omelette begins to set, sprinkle half the zucchini and cheese on top. Continue cooking over a low heat until the cheese has melted. Fold the omelette in half, cut into 2 and serve with the cucumber. Repeat to make a second omelette.

sautéed wild mushrooms and walnuts

butter	2 tbsp
walnut oil	3 tbsp
wild mushrooms	6 ounces, wiped and cut into about ½-inch slices
walnuts	2 ounces, chopped
Little Gem lettuce	1, trimmed and chopped
soft goat's cheese	3½ ounces, cut into small cubes

For breakfast, brunch, or even a light supper, this is a great recipe for 2 people. It is rich in mono-unsaturated fats from the walnuts and walnut oil, which help eliminate cholesterol and protect the heart and circulation. Easily digested and perfect as a post-detox dish when you are returning to normal meals.

Melt the butter gently with the walnut oil in a large frying pan over a low heat. Add the mushrooms and walnuts, cover the pan and simmer gently for 10 minutes. Arrange the lettuce on 2 serving plates. Using a slotted spoon, remove the mushrooms and walnuts from the pan and arrange over the lettuce. Scatter on the goat's cheese and top with the juices from the frying pan. Serve immediately.

colcannon

white cabbage	8 ounces
potatoes	1 pound, peeled and sliced
carrot	1, small, scrubbed and diced
turnip	1, small, thoroughly washed and thinly sliced
2 percent milk	1 cup
leek	1, small, cleaned, trimmed and finely sliced
eggs	2

An Irish chef on my radio program once gave "the definitive" recipe for colcannon. For the next three hours the phone rang as members of the London Irish community claimed they all had a better recipe. However, this is my favorite version, stolen from my wife's family in County Cavan. The sulphur in the cabbage, the vitamin A in the carrot, the minerals in the turnip and the anti-bacterial chemicals in the leeks are what I believe explain the sweet complexion for which Irish girls are famous.

Boil the cabbage until just tender, chop finely, then reserve until required. Meanwhile, boil the potatoes, carrot and turnip together until tender and mash coarsely. Heat the milk in a saucepan, add the leek and simmer gently until tender. Drain the leek, reserving the milk, and mash the cooked leek with the cooked cabbage into the potato mixture. Add enough of the leek milk to make a firm mash. Transfer to a casserole dish and broil under a preheated broiler until golden on top. Meanwhile, poach the eggs and serve on top of the vegetable mixture.

cinnamon toast with figs

eggs	4
ground cinnamon	2 tsp
whole-wheat bread	4 medium slices
butter	6 tbsp
dark brown sugar	2 tbsp
fresh figs	4, halved lengthwise

What a wonderful start to a leisurely day – and a great radiance boost too! The eggs in this delicious recipe contain iron, B vitamins and protein and there are cleansing essential oils in the cinnamon. Added to this, there's the ultimate pleasure of combining those delicious flavors with fresh figs, known since ancient times as one of nature's great skin foods.

Beat the eggs with half the cinnamon in a large bowl. Cut the bread into thick fingers. Melt the butter in a frying pan. Dip the bread in the egg mixture and fry in the butter on both sides until golden. Sprinkle with the brown sugar and the rest of the cinnamon. Serve with the figs on the side.

radiance teabread

egg	1
camomile tea	1 cup made with 5 teabags and allowed to cool completely before the teabags are removed
dried dates	1 pound, chopped
soft brown sugar	1 scant cup
self-rising flour	1½ cups

The calming effect of camomile, and the iron and fibre in the dates make this bread a delicious and extremely healthy snack.

Beat the egg. Put all the other ingredients in a large mixing bowl, add the beaten egg, and mix well. Let stand for at least 6 hours. Preheat the oven to 350°F. Line an 8-inch loaf pan with waxed paper. Pour the mixture into the pan and bake in the preheated oven for 30 minutes. Turn out onto a wire rack and leave to cool.

energy teabread

Earl Grey tea	1 cup, made with 5 teabags and allowed to cool
dried dates	1 pound chopped into raisin-size pieces
turbinado or raw sugar	1 cup
egg	1, beaten
self-rising flour	1½ cups

People often think treats like this are sinful, but this certainly isn't. One generous slice will be a huge boost to your flagging energy, and thanks to the dates, provides plenty of disease-fighting anti-oxidants.

Mix all the ingredients together and let stand, covered with a clean dish towel, for at least 6 hours. Preheat the oven to 350°F. Pour the mixture into an 8-inch loaf pan lined with waxed paper. Bake in the preheated oven for 30 minutes. Turn out of the pan and leave to cool on a wire rack.

real swiss muesli

organic low-salt unsweetened muesli	12 heaped tbsp
apple juice	about 2 cups
live natural yogurt	about 2 cups

The slow-release energy from the oats in the muesli makes them perfect for breakfast or brunch as they help keep your blood sugar on an even keel for several hours. This means you avoid those mid-morning sugar cravings. This recipe makes enough for 2 people.

Put the muesli into 2 bowls. Pour on the apple juice – don't worry if the mixture seems very runny; the cereal will expand. Stir in the yogurt and leave in the refrigerator overnight.

porridge with cinnamon and dried fruits

uncooked oats	2 average cups
2 percent milk	2 average cups
water	2 average cups
mixed dried fruits	⅔ cup
ground cinnamon	2 level tsp

This has all the energy and blood-sugar benefits of the oats, plus the huge anti-oxidant and protective value of the fruits.

Put the oats, milk and water into a saucepan. Bring to the boil and simmer for 5 minutes or according to the package instructions, stirring regularly. While it's cooking, cut the dried fruits into evenly sized pieces, about as big as a little fingernail. When the porridge is cooked, stir in the fruit and 1 tsp of cinnamon. Cover and let stand for 2 minutes. Serve with the remaining cinnamon sprinkled on top and extra milk, if desired.

scrambled eggs with smoked salmon

unsalted butter	4 tbsp
2 percent milk	½ cup
eggs	8
smoked salmon	4 ounces of trimmings – you don't need expensive slices – cut into fine slivers
black pepper	to taste
chives	10, snipped
toast or rustic bread	to serve

Put the butter and milk in a large, preferably nonstick, frying pan and heat gently until the butter has melted. Remove the pan from the heat and crack in the eggs. Gently break up the yolks, but don't amalgamate them fully with the egg white. Return to a low heat. Using a wooden spatula, push the mixture regularly from the edges to the middle of the pan, again leaving some definition between the yolks and whites. When the eggs are almost as firm as you like them – the heat of the pan will continue the cooking process for several minutes – remove the pan from the heat and stir in the smoked salmon. Season to taste with freshly ground black pepper and serve with the chives sprinkled on top and accompanied by toast or chunks of rustic bread.

mushrooms on whole-wheat toast

well-flavored mushrooms	10 ounces
unsalted butter	6 tbsp
parsley	4 large sprigs, leaves finely chopped
whole-wheat bread	4 slices

Wipe and slice the mushrooms. Melt the butter gently in a small frying pan and add the chopped parsley. Sauté the mushrooms over a low heat until the juices run, about 10 minutes. Just before they're cooked, toast the bread and serve with the mushroom mixture piled on top.

buckwheat crêpes

butter	4 tbsp
2 percent milk	1½ cups
buckwheat flour	¾ cup
organic all-purpose flour	¾ cup, sifted
salt	¼ tsp
eggs	4
canola oil	for frying
pumpkin seeds	3 tbsp
lemons	juice of 2, large
honey	4 tbsp

Crêpes always seem like an indulgence, but the rutin and natural chemicals in buckwheat ensure that energizing oxygen nutrients get to where they need to be and protect the tiniest blood vessels under the skin, helping to prevent problems like thread veins, pimples and other skin blemishes.

Melt the butter and stir it into the milk. Put the flours and salt together in a food processor. With the motor running continuously, pour in the milk and butter mixture. With the motor still on, add the eggs one at a time until you have a smooth batter. Let the mixture rest in the refrigerator for at least 1 hour.

Brush a crêpe pan or small frying pan with a little oil and heat over a medium heat until the oil is smoking. Pour in a ladleful of batter, tilting the pan to spread it evenly. When the underside is golden, turn the crêpe – or toss it if you feel like showing off – and cook for a further 1–2 minutes. Slide the crêpe onto a paper towel and keep warm while you repeat with the rest of the batter.

Dry-fry the pumpkin seeds for 2 minutes, until just turning colour. Drizzle each crêpe with the lemon juice and honey, fold in

savory toasties

unsalted butter	for spreading
whole-wheat bread	4 thick slices
tomatoes	2, sliced
green bell pepper	½, seeded and very finely chopped
onion	1, small, very finely chopped
paprika	2 pinches
Gruyère cheese	2 heaped tbsp, grated

Preheat the oven to 450°F. Butter the bread, arrange the slices of tomato on top and cook in the preheated oven for 7 minutes. Put the chopped pepper and onion on top of the tomatoes with a pinch of paprika on each slice. Sprinkle the cheese on top and return to the oven until the cheese is bubbling, about 5 minutes.

poached kippers and tomatoes

kippers	2 pairs, undyed
tomatoes	4
unsalted butter	4 tbsp
lemon	juice of ½
parsley	1 heaped tbsp finely chopped leaves

Even though kippers are salty, they're a great source of energy-producing protein and also provide some iodine, which is essential for the effective action of the thyroid. The fish oils in kippers are also an anti-inflammatory and vital for heart protection.

Bring a large shallow saucepan of water to the boil. Add the kippers and tomatoes and simmer for about 5 minutes. Meanwhile, cream the butter and stir in the lemon juice and parsley and reserve. Remove the kippers and tomatoes from the water with a slotted spoon. Pat the kippers dry with kitchen paper. Slip the skins off the tomatoes. Serve with a lump of the prepared butter on each kipper.

english breakfast the healthy way

mushrooms	2, large, wiped
bacon	4 extra-lean strips
traditional sausages	4
tomatoes	2, halved widthwise
eggs	4
whole-wheat toast	to serve

I'm convinced that one factor in the epidemic of chronic fatigue is people's failure to eat a proper breakfast. The traditional English breakfast has been so criticized that rather than eat it at home, many people sneak off to a café on their way to work. My old friend and first of the super chefs, Anton Mosimann, taught me the egg trick.

Preheat the broiler and line the broiler pan with foil. Put the mushrooms, bacon, sausages, and tomatoes on the broiler pan and put under the broiler. While they're cooking, put a large plate on top of a saucepan of simmering water. When the plate is really hot, break the eggs onto it and leave to cook. Serve this traditional breakfast with good whole-wheat toast.

drinks

In all detox plans, maintaining a high fluid intake is essential if you are to achieve the overall cleansing benefits you're aiming for. These simple recipes for juices and smoothies are included here for two reasons: first, to help you cope with your reduced calorie intake during the detox programs, and second, to get you into the habit of using and enjoying these super-nutrient drinks as part of your normal life.

I recommend that you make your own juices from fresh, organic produce. It's not as difficult as you might think, but this really is the moment to invest in a good juicer or blender for your kitchen. As with everything, buy the best you can afford.

For juicing, most produce only needs washing and cutting into small enough pieces to fit into the machine. There's normally no need to peel or remove the core, but obviously you must take out any pits. Thick skins, like those on mangoes and pineapples, usually need to be removed. There are no rules, just experiment with whatever you have in stock to find your favourite combos. Once you get the hang of it, you'll be hooked!

carrot, apple, and celery juice

carrots	3, large, trimmed – and peeled if not organic
apples	2, quartered
celery	2 stalks

Put all the ingredients in a blender or liquidizer and whiz together until smooth.

yogurt and strawberry smoothie

live natural yogurt	1 pint (2 cups)
strawberries	21 ounces
cilantro	6 large stalks

Put all the ingredients in a blender and whiz together until smooth.

apple, peanut, and banana smoothie

apples	3, quartered and juiced
bananas	2
smooth peanut butter	2 tbsp
soy milk	1¼ cups

An excellent start to anybody's day thanks to the high-energy value of the bananas and peanuts. This smoothie also provides the health benefits of soy milk, which helps protect against hormonal swings, osteoporosis, and breast cancer.

Put all the ingredients in a blender and whiz together until smooth.

tomato juice with green onions

tomatoes	8, large
green onions	2 fat bulbs, trimmed
basil	4 large sprigs
oregano	6 large sprigs

Roughly chop the tomatoes and green onions and put into a blender with the leaves from the basil and oregano. Whiz until smooth.

carrot, apple, and beet juice

carrots	3, large, trimmed and peeled if not organic
apples	2, quartered
beets	2, small, raw with leaves

It's the high natural sugar content of the beets that makes this juice an energy booster. But there's an added bonus in the form of the skin-friendly vitamin A in the carrots.

Put all the ingredients in a blender and whiz together until smooth.

tomato juice, celery, and celery leaf blend

plum tomatoes	6, large, ripe
celery	2 stalks, with leaves
lemon	juice of 1
Tabasco (optional)	a dash

Put the tomatoes, celery, and lemon juice in a blender or food processor and blend until smooth. Season to taste with the Tabasco sauce, if using.

orange juice and almond blend

oranges	4 large, juiced
ground almonds	4 tbsp

Simply mix the two ingredients together and whisk with a fork.

kiwi and pineapple juice

kiwi fruit	4, ripe, peeled
pineapple	1, top removed

Just cut the fruit into pieces and juice. Some of the heavy-duty juicers will cope with fruit with a tough skin like pineapples. Check your machine's instructions.

yogurt and mango smoothie

live natural yogurt	1½ cups
mango	1, large, ripe, peeled and cubed

Put the ingredients in a blender and whiz until smooth.

apple, kiwi, pear, and celery juice

apples	3, quartered
kiwi fruit	3, ripe, peeled
pears	2
celery	2 stalks, with leaves

Put all the ingredients in a blender and whiz until smooth.

grape, pear, apple, and pineapple juice

seedless blue or purple grapes	1 cup
pears	3
apples	3, quartered
pineapple	½, large

Put all the ingredients in a blender and whiz until smooth.

berry smoothie

mixed fresh berries	⅔ cup, hulled
live natural yogurt	1½ cups
lemon	zest of ½
ground cinnamon	½ level tsp
mint	2 sprigs

Put all the ingredients into a blender and whiz until smooth. Serve garnished with a sprig of fresh mint.

yogurt and prune smoothie

live natural yogurt	2 cups
prunes	12, pitted

Put the ingredients in a blender and whiz until smooth.

ginger tea

Add 1 inch fresh grated gingerroot to a mug of boiling water. Cover and let stand for 5 minutes. Strain, add 1 tsp of honey, and sip slowly.

parsley tea

Put 2 heaped tbsp of chopped fresh parsley into a pitcher. Add 2 cups of boiling water, cover and leave to stand for 10 minutes. Strain, cool and keep covered in the refrigerator.

radiance juice

dessert apple	1, large, quartered
orange	1, peeled, but with as much pith as possible
carrots	2, large, trimmed – and peeled if not organic
gingerroot	1 inch, peeled and sliced

This zingy juice full of vitamins A and C from the carrots and orange, soluble fiber for regular digestive function from the apple, and stimulating gingerole from the ginger will do more for your skin than a dozen pots of expensive cream. All these nutrients will improve the circulation, helping to carry health-giving nutrients directly to the skin.

Put all the ingredients in a blender and whiz until smooth.

radiance lemonade

carrot	1, large, trimmed – and peeled if not organic
radishes	10, trimmed
apple	1, quartered
beet	1, trimmed
lemons	juice and finely grated zest of 2
naturally sparkling mineral water (optional)	up to 1¼ cups

Vitamin A is essential for healthy, radiant skin and you'll get it in abundance from the carrots in this juice. The bonus comes from the radishes; their natural constituents stimulate the cleansing function of the liver, making this the perfect juice when you've been a bit over-indulgent or your digestive system seems slightly sluggish.

Juice the first 4 ingredients. Add the lemon juice and zest. If you want a longer, fizzy drink, add the mineral water.

soy, blueberry, and strawberry smoothie

blueberries	½ cup
strawberries	6, large
soy milk	1½ cups

Blueberries and strawberries on their own are super radiance boosters, but adding soy milk brings extra benefits. The natural plant hormones in soy help to regulate the hormonal seesaw of the menstrual cycle and also prevent some of the symptoms of menopause, making this smoothie extremely female-friendly.

Put all the ingredients in a blender and whiz until smooth.

mango and soy milk smoothie

mango	1, large, ripe, cubed
soy milk	1½ cups

Put the ingredients in a blender and whiz until smooth.

yogurt, papaya, and kiwi smoothie

live natural yogurt	2½ cups
papaya	1, peeled, seeded, cubed
kiwi fruit	2, peeled and cubed

Put all the ingredients in a blender and whiz until smooth.

kiwi and passion fruit smoothie

passion fruit	4
mascarpone cheese	1 cup
2 percent milk	⅓ cup
kiwi fruit	3, peeled and cut into chunks

Cut the passion fruit in half widthwise and rub through a sieve to extract all the juice. Discard the seeds. Put the passion fruit juice with the rest of the ingredients in a blender or food processor and whiz until smooth. Alternatively, use an immersion blender.

mango, kiwi, and pineapple juice

This exotic juice is packed full of vitamins A, C and E, healing enzymes and a massive amount of natural plant chemicals.

mango	1, large, ripe, pitted
kiwi fruit	4
pineapple	1, top and peel removed

Cut the ingredients into chunks, put in a blender and whiz until smooth.

carrot and beet juice

carrots	4, trimmed – and peeled if not organic
beets	4, preferably with leaves
basil	3 large sprigs

Put all the ingredients in a blender and whiz until smooth.

lunches and dinners

mixed vegetable stir-fry with rice

sesame oil	2 tbsp
canola oil	2 tbsp
carrots	2, in julienne strips
broccoli	12 small florets
celery	2 stalks, finely sliced
green onions	4, cut diagonally
snow peas	¾ cup, quartered
baby corn	¾ cup, in ½-inch chunks
fresh peas	½ cup
basmati rice	⅔ cup
very veggie stock (see recipe, page 227)	about 1 quart
light soy sauce	2 tsp

With such a wide variety of vegetables, this is an amazingly protective dish full of resistance-boosting nutrients.

Heat the oils in a preheated wok or large frying pan. Add the vegetables and cook over a medium heat for 5 minutes, stirring continuously, until just al dente. Meanwhile, cook the rice in a saucepan of boiling water according to the package instructions. Pour the stock into the vegetables and boil rapidly until most of the liquid is absorbed. Add the soy sauce, mix thoroughly, and serve the vegetables over the rice.

home-made chicken liver pâté

unsalted butter	5 tbsp
onion	1, very finely chopped
garlic	2 cloves, very finely chopped
chicken livers	1 pound, fresh or frozen, washed and with membranes removed
light cream	3 tbsp
tomato purée	1 tbsp
brandy	2 tbsp
bay leaves	3
parsley	1 tbsp freshly chopped leaves

This may seem an unhealthy inclusion for a detox book, but it's a far cry from commercially made pâtés. Yes, it does contain butter, cream, and brandy, but it's also full of iron, B vitamins – especially B12 – and all the cleansing properties of garlic, onions, and parsley. Indulge.

Melt half the butter in a large frying pan and sauté the onion and garlic gently for 3 minutes. Add the chicken livers and continue cooking gently for 5 minutes, stirring continuously, until soft but not browned. Transfer to a bowl and mash thoroughly with a fork. Pour in the cream, tomato purée, and brandy and mix again, adding more cream if the mixture seems too thick. Spoon into a 2-cup terrine or other suitable dish and refrigerate.

When the pâté is cool and set, melt the rest of the butter in a small saucepan. Place the bay leaves on the pâté, sprinkle the parsley on top, pour over the melted butter and return to the refrigerator until the butter is set.

pasta with lettuce pesto

A wonderfully healthy pasta, providing energy, calcium and protein, plus calming natural chemicals to help you unwind and sleep.

fusilli	1 pound
radicchio	1 large head, washed
pine nuts	
extra-virgin olive oil	4 tbsp
Parmesan cheese	4 tbsp, freshly grated
lettuce	1 small handful, leaves roughly torn

Cook the pasta in a large saucepan of boiling water according to the package instructions. Meanwhile, put the radicchio, pine nuts and half the oil into a food processor and whiz until smooth. With the machine running, add the rest of the oil in a gentle stream. When thoroughly blended, pour into a bowl and stir in the cheese and lettuce. Stir the pesto into the pasta and serve.

grilled chicken breast on iceberg lettuce

chicken breasts	4, skinless, boneless and flattened slightly
lime	juice of 1
extra-virgin olive oil	2 tbsp
garlic	1 clove, finely chopped
tarragon	4 sprigs
Iceberg lettuce	1

Put the chicken breasts into a large, shallow dish. Mix the lime juice, olive oil and garlic together in a separate bowl and pour over the chicken. Add the tarragon and stir until the chicken is well coated in the marinade. Cover with plastic wrap and refrigerate for at least 1 hour.

Preheat the broiler. Drain the chicken, reserving the marinade. Put the chicken on the broiler pan and broil for 15 minutes, turning once. Meanwhile, shred the lettuce and thoroughly heat the rest of the marinade in a small saucepan. Serve the chicken on the lettuce, drizzled with the marinade.

mushrooms with radicchio and chicory

unsalted butter	4 tbsp
mushrooms	4, large, wiped and peeled
chicory	2 heads
whole-wheat bread	4 thick slices
radicchio	1 bunch

Heat the butter in a large heavy-bottomed pan until soft. Add the mushrooms, cover the pan and cook over a medium heat for 10 minutes. Remove from the heat and transfer to a foil-lined broiler pan. Broil under a low flame until the juices begin to run. Brush the chicory leaves with the butter from the mushrooms, and put under the broiler until wilted. Divide the bread between 4 serving plates, arrange the radicchio on top, the charred chicory around the edges, then add the mushrooms and serve.

deviled sardines

fresh sardines	4, cleaned
Dijon mustard	2 tbsp
cayenne pepper	1 tsp
whole-wheat bread	4 slices
tomatoes	2, sliced
lemon	1, quartered

I cannot emphasize too often the importance of oily fish. They're a natural anti-inflammatory and essential during pregnancy and breastfeeding for the growing baby's brain development. They are also the richest source of vitamin D – needed to turn calcium into strong bones.

Preheat the broiler and line the broiler pan with foil. Make diagonal cuts in the sardines and rub with the mustard. Sprinkle the cayenne pepper on both sides. Broil for 5 minutes, turning once. Meanwhile, toast the bread. Serve the sardines with the toast, tomatoes, and lemon quarters.

special welsh rarebit

medium Cheddar cheese	1½ cups, grated
whole milk	3 tbsp
Worcestershire sauce	1 tsp
Dijon mustard	1 tsp
paprika	1 pinch
parsley	2 tsp freshly chopped leaves
whole-wheat bread	4 thick slices

A slice of processed cheese grilled on a piece of bread isn't a Welsh rarebit. Try this recipe instead – it contains lots of healing nutrients, has a great flavor and only takes a few minutes.

Preheat the grill and line the grill pan with foil. Mix the cheese and milk together. Add the Worcestershire sauce, mustard, paprika and half the parsley and stir again until completely combined. Toast the bread on one side, turn it over and arrange the cheese mixture on top. Return to the grill and cook until the cheese bubbles. Serve with the extra parsley scattered on top.

ratatouille

extra-virgin olive oil	6 tbsp
onions	2, large, finely chopped
garlic	4 cloves, finely chopped
green bell peppers	2, large, seeded and finely chopped
eggplant	1, large, finely cubed
chopped tomatoes	1 x 15-ounce can

Heat the olive oil and sauté the onions and garlic gently for 5 minutes in a large saucepan. Add the peppers and eggplant and continue to sauté for a further 5 minutes. Add the tomatoes, cover the pan, and simmer gently for 30 minutes.

baked stuffed trout

extra-virgin olive oil	4 tbsp
onion	1, large, finely chopped
garlic	2 cloves, finely chopped
butter beans	1 cup, canned or cooked, mashed
fresh spinach	6 ounces, thoroughly washed and roughly torn
lake or brook trout	4, cleaned
dry white wine	8 ounces
unsalted butter	5 tbsp
lemon	1, large, sliced

Trout is another wonderful oily fish. Need I say more?

Preheat the oven to 425°F. Heat the olive oil in a saucepan and sauté the onion and garlic gently for 5 minutes. Drain off any excess oil. Mix the onion and garlic into the mashed beans and spinach. Cut 4 pieces of foil large enough to make a parcel around each fish. Lay a fish on each piece of foil and fill each fish cavity with the bean and spinach mixture. Pour a quarter of the wine over each. Dot with the butter and top with a slice of lemon. Fold the foil over and tuck in the ends. Place the parcels on baking sheets and cook for 20 minutes.

veggie curry with rice

extra-virgin olive oil	6 tbsp
onion	1, large, finely sliced
garlic	2 cloves, finely chopped
red chile	1, small, seeded and finely chopped
gingerroot	½-inch, peeled and grated
green Thai curry paste	1 heaped tbsp
cauliflower	10 florets
carrots	3, in fine julienne strips
new potatoes	2, in ½-inch cubes
parsnip	1, peeled, in ½-inch cubes
turnip	1, peeled, in ½-inch cubes
very veggie stock (see recipe, page 227)	2 cups
coconut milk	1½ cups
basmati rice	⅔ cup

At first sight, you may not think of curry as part of a healthy detox plan, but you'd be wrong. Apart from the cleansing and health-promoting vegetables, the turmeric in curry paste is a valuable anti-cancer spice.

Heat the oil in a large saucepan and gently soften the onion, garlic, chile and ginger for 5 minutes. Add the curry paste and stir until completely combined. Add the cauliflower, carrots, potatoes, parsnip, and turnip and stir continuously for a further 10 minutes. Pour in the stock and coconut milk and simmer for 40 minutes until all the vegetables are tender.

Meanwhile, cook the rice according to the package instructions. Serve the rice with the vegetable curry on top.

tuna and cottage-cheese stuffed tomatoes

beefsteak tomatoes	8, large, sliced widthwise, membranes and seeds removed
tuna	1 6-ounce can, in olive oil, drained
cottage cheese	1 8-ounce tub
capers	2 tbsp, soaked in milk for 5 mins, then drained
chives	10 snipped, 4 left whole
black pepper	to taste

Put the tomatoes into a wide, shallow dish. Mix the drained tuna, cottage cheese, capers, and snipped chives together in a bowl. Season to taste with black pepper. Pile the tuna and cheese mixture into the tomato hollows. Garnish with the remaining chives and serve.

stir-fried tofu with vegetables and noodles

lime	juice of 1
mango	1, peeled and finely cubed
Tabasco sauce	½ tsp
garlic	2 cloves, finely chopped
tofu	9 ounces, drained and cubed
onion	1, finely chopped
extra-virgin olive oil	2 tbsp
instant noodles	
kale	6 ounces, finely chopped
beansprouts	8 ounces

Most carnivores eat far too much meat. Good meat, preferably organic, in modest quantities, is great food if you like it. But too much has been linked to bowel cancer, raised cholesterol, and high blood pressure. Here's your chance to use tofu, a soy product that's rich in natural plant hormones and extremely healthful.

Preheat the oven to 425°F. Mix the lime, mango, Tabasco sauce, and half the garlic together in a bowl. Put the tofu into a shallow dish, add the marinade and stir to coat. Cover with plastic wrap and refrigerate for 30 minutes. Transfer the tofu and marinade to the preheated oven and cook for 20 minutes.

Meanwhile, sauté the onion and remaining garlic in the oil in a wok or large frying pan for 5 minutes. In another pan, cook the noodles according to the package instructions, usually 2–3 minutes. Add the kale and beansprouts to the onion mixture and stir until just wilted. Drain the noodles, add to the wok, and cook for a further 2 minutes. Add the tofu with its marinade and stir gently before serving.

pasta all'aglio e olio

spaghettini	1 pound
extra-virgin olive oil	6 tbsp
garlic	3 cloves, peeled and crushed with the flat blade of a broad knife
Parmesan cheese	4 tbsp, freshly grated
basil	6 large sprigs, leaves removed and finely torn

This dish is great for both its energy-giving and health-boosting properties. The garlic lowers cholesterol, reduces blood pressure and makes blood less likely to clot, as well as being antibacterial and antifungal.

Cook the pasta according to the package instructions. Meanwhile, heat the olive oil in a saucepan, add the garlic and cook gently until just beginning to turn brown. Remove the garlic with a slotted spoon and discard. Pour the hot oil over the pasta and mix thoroughly. Stir in the Parmesan cheese and mix again. Finally, stir in the basil leaves and serve immediately.

broiled salmon steak

salmon steaks	4
extra-virgin olive oil	6 tbsp
black pepper	to taste
tarragon	8 sprigs; 4 whole, 4 with the leaves removed and finely chopped
unsalted butter	5 tbsp, softened

Put the salmon steaks into a wide casserole dish. Pour over the olive oil and season to taste with freshly ground black pepper. Add the whole tarragon sprigs. Turn the salmon over carefully in the dish to marinate, cover with plastic wrap and refrigerate for 1 hour. Meanwhile, mix the chopped tarragon into the softened butter and put it into the refrigerator to harden.

Preheat the broiler to high and line the broiler pan with foil. Remove the salmon from the marinade, leaving some of the oil clinging. Broil the fish for 6–7 minutes, turning once. Serve with the tarragon butter on top.

baked leeks with cheese and eggs

baby leeks	16, cleaned and trimmed, but with most of the green parts retained if they're tender
light cream	¾ cup
eggs	3
Emmental cheese	4 ounces, grated
salt and black pepper	to taste
parsley	3 tbsp finely chopped leaves

Preheat the oven to 400°F. Put the leeks into a saucepan of boiling water and simmer for 5 minutes. Drain carefully and place in an oblong casserole. Whisk the cream, eggs, and half the cheese together. Season to taste. Pour the mixture over the leeks and sprinkle the rest of the cheese over the top. Bake in the preheated oven for 15 minutes, until the cheese is golden and beginning to bubble. Serve sprinkled with the parsley.

falafel

This classic Middle Eastern dish is another meat-free treat, with no saturated fat or cholesterol, lots of calcium, and plenty of protein.

chickpeas	2 x 14-ounce cans, drained and rinsed
extra-virgin olive oil	4 tbsp
onion	1, large, finely chopped
garlic	2 cloves, finely chopped
parsley	4 tbsp finely chopped leaves
allspice	5 tsp
baking powder	½ tsp
canola oil	about 1 cup
Iceberg lettuce	1, shredded

Put the chickpeas and olive oil into a blender and whiz until smooth. Add the onion, garlic, parsley, allspice, and baking powder and whiz again. Transfer the mixture to a bowl and form into small burger-type shapes, about 1 inch across. Place on a flat plate and refrigerate for 30 minutes.

Heat the canola oil in a large frying pan and fry the falafel for about 2 minutes on each side. Drain on paper towels. Serve on a bed of Iceberg lettuce.

game hen casserole with red cabbage

Game, is low in fat, but rich in iron and B vitamins. With the red cabbage, you get all the traditional protection and health promotion of this king of vegetables.

for the casserole

Cornish game hens	2
garlic	6 cloves, sliced
lemon	1
thyme	4 large sprigs
extra-virgin olive oil	2 tbsp
onion	1, finely sliced
carrots	2, sliced

for the red cabbage 4 tbsp

onion	1, finely sliced
garlic	2 cloves, finely chopped
red cabbage	1, finely sliced
cider vinegar	4 tbsp
brown sugar	1 tbsp

Preheat the oven to 350°F. Make several incisions into the flesh of the hens and insert the sliced garlic. Rub the skins with the lemon and put the thyme inside the cavities. Heat the oil in a heavy-based metal casserole and sauté the onion and carrots for 5 minutes, then remove from the casserole and reserve. Add the hens and brown on all sides. Add the reserved onions and carrots. Cover and cook in the preheated oven for 45 minutes, until the juices run clear when a skewer is inserted into the thickest part of the thigh.

Meanwhile, cook the cabbage. Heat the oil in a saucepan and sauté the onion and garlic gently. Stir in the cabbage and add the vinegar and sugar. Transfer to a metal casserole dish, cover and cook with the hens for the last 30 minutes of cooking time.

Serve the hens with the red cabbage and with the onion and carrots, which will have made a wonderfully flavored purée.

couscous with vegetables

dried fruit	4 ounces, mixed raisins and apricots
olive oil	4 tbsp
onion	1, finely sliced
leek	1, cleaned, trimmed and finely sliced
carrots	2, diced
celery	2 stalks, finely sliced
mushrooms	4 ounces, finely sliced
couscous	1 pound

Snip the apricots to the size of the raisins. Heat the oil in a saucepan and sauté the onion gently until soft. Add the other vegetables and the dried fruit, cover, and cook gently until tender – about 15 minutes. Add water if it seems to be drying out.

Meanwhile, bring 2 cups of water to the boil in a large saucepan. Add the couscous, reduce the heat and cook for 1 minute, stirring continuously. Remove from the heat, cover and let stand for 5 minutes until all the water is absorbed. Stir in the vegetables and dried fruit and serve.

organic beef stew with vegetables

If you're going to eat beef occasionally, splash out and go organic. It tastes better, and contains less saturated fat and much more of the health-promoting fat CLA (conjugated linoleic acid), which is essential for the breakdown of other fats.

canola oil	4 tbsp
onion	1, finely sliced
garlic	2 cloves, peeled and finely chopped
organic all-purpose flour	3 heaped tbsp
herbs de Provence	1 level tbsp
lean organic top round or bottom round steak	1 pound, cubed
very veggie stock (see recipe, page 227)	1 quart
carrots	2, finely sliced
turnip	1, cubed
parsnip	1, in julienne strips
celery	2 stalks, sliced
bay leaves	2
ked rice or mashed potatoes	to serve

Heat the oil gently in a pan and sauté the onion and garlic for 5 minutes. Mix the flour and herbs de Provence together in a bowl and use to coat the meat. Add the meat to the pan and stir until browned on all sides. Pour in the stock, the rest of the vegetables, and the bay leaves. Cover and simmer for about 1½ hours until the meat is tender, adding water if it looks as if it's drying out. Remove and discard the bay leaves and serve with rice or mashed potatoes.

spinach with yogurt

baby spinach leaves	2 pounds
unsalted butter	2 tbsp
pumpkin seeds	3 tbsp
live natural yogurt	⅔ cup

Wash the spinach and put into a saucepan with only the water clinging to it. Add the butter and pumpkin seeds. Cover and cook over a very low heat until the spinach is wilted, about 7 minutes. Drain, cool slightly, and chop roughly. Stir in the yogurt and serve.

broiled marinated fish

extra-virgin olive oil	4 tbsp
onion	1, small, very finely chopped
lime	juice of 1
mixed parsley, fennel fronds, dill, coriander and tarragon	4 tbsp, finely chopped
fish fillets, any variety	4
Cheddar cheese	2 tbsp, grated

Mix the oil, onion, lime juice, and herbs together in a large, shallow dish. Add the fish and coat thoroughly in the marinade. Cover with plastic wrap and refrigerate for at least 30 minutes.

Preheat the broiler to high. Drain the fish, reserving the marinade. Place the fish in the broiler pan and brush each side with the marinade. Broil for up to 5 minutes on each side, depending on the thickness of the fish. Sprinkle over the cheese and broil for a further 1 minute, until the cheese bubbles. Serve immediately.

mixed cabbage, leek, and green onions

walnut oil	3 tbsp
sesame oil	3 tbsp
Savoy cabbage	1, finely shredded
leeks	3, cleaned, trimmed and finely sliced
green onions	6 plump, roughly chopped
carrots	2, grated
sesame seeds	2 tbsp
light soy or hoisin sauce	2 tbsp

This is the ultimate detoxing and health-boosting vegetable dish. Heart-protective, artery-friendly, and anti-cancer nutrients abound. There's also lots of sulphur, so it's great for blemished skins.

Heat the oils in a large frying pan or a preheated wok. Add the vegetables and stir-fry until soft, stirring continuously, for about 10 minutes. Add the sesame seeds and soy or hoisin sauce and heat through for a further minute.

chicken jalfrezi

canola oil	4 tbsp
cumin seeds	1 tsp
garlic	3 cloves, finely chopped
gingerroot	1½ inches, peeled and grated
turmeric	1 tsp
green Thai curry paste	2 level tbsp
chicken breasts	1 pound, 12 ounces skinless, cut into thin strips along the grain
red chiles	2, seeded and finely chopped
orange bell pepper	1, seeded and cubed
tomatoes	1 x 8-ounce can
coconut milk	4 ounces
coriander	2 tbsp freshly chopped leaves
garam masala	2 tsp
cooked rice	to serve

Heat the oil in a large frying pan or preheated wok. Add the cumin seeds, garlic, ginger, turmeric, curry paste and 1 tsp of water. Add the chicken pieces, stir to coat in the spices and cook for 2 minutes. Add the chiles, pepper and tomatoes and simmer for 10 minutes. Pour in the coconut milk and add the coriander. Simmer for a further 5 minutes or until the chicken is tender. Add the garam masala and cook for 2 minutes. Serve with rice.

baked cod with sesame seeds

cod steaks	4
eggs	2, beaten
sesame seeds	4 ounces

It's the energy boost from the sesame seeds that makes this simple dish different. Like all seeds, sesame seeds are rich in vitamin E.

Preheat the oven to 325°F. Dip the fish in the eggs, then the sesame seeds. Put on a large baking sheet and bake in the preheated oven for 20 minutes.

bulgur with eggplant

bulgur wheat	1 cup
olive oil	8 tbsp
onion	1, large, finely chopped
eggplants	2, cubed
ground coriander	3 tsp
ground cumin	3 tsp
flaked almonds	150g
raisins	110g

Simmer the bulgur wheat in twice its volume of water until most of the water has been absorbed, about 10 minutes. Set aside. Meanwhile, heat the oil and fry the onion until golden. Add the eggplant and continue frying until both are crisp, adding more oil if necessary. Add the coriander and cumin and cook for 1 minute, stirring continuously. Reduce the heat, add the almonds and raisins, and cook for 2 minutes or until the almonds are golden. Stir in the bulgur wheat, drained if necessary, and heat through for about 1 minute.

pasta noodles with broccoli

broccoli	12 ounces, fresh, cut into small florets — frozen won't work
egg linguine	1 pound
olive oil	4 tbsp
garlic	2 large cloves, finely chopped
anchovy paste	1 level tsp
red chile	½, seeded and very finely chopped
Parmesan cheese	4 tbsp, freshly grated

Blanch the broccoli florets in a saucepan of boiling water for 5 minutes. Remove from the water and reserve. Add the pasta to the water and cook according to the package instructions. Meanwhile, heat the oil in a large frying pan and add the garlic, anchovy paste and chile. Add the broccoli and continue cooking, stirring continuously, for 5 minutes. Drain the pasta. Pour the garlic, anchovy and chile mixture over and serve immediately with the Parmesan cheese.

salmon in a parcel

salmon fillets	4
extra-virgin olive oil	4 tbsp
tarragon	4 sprigs
parsley	4 tbsp freshly chopped leaves
capers	2 tbsp, rinsed and chopped
lemon	4 slices

Preheat the oven to 400°F. Cut 4 pieces of foil each large enough to make a parcel around a fillet. Put the fish onto the foil and divide the olive oil, tarragon, parsley, and capers between them. Top each with a slice of lemon. Fold the foil over and tuck in the ends. Place the parcels on baking sheets and bake in the preheated oven for 20 minutes.

pan-fried liver

canola oil	4 tbsp
unsalted butter	4 tbsp
onion	1, large, finely chopped
unsmoked bacon	4 thin strips, cut in 2 lengthwise
calves' liver	1 pound, 9 ounces, thinly sliced
sherry	5 tbsp
parsley	4 tbsp finely chopped leaves

Liver is the organ that stores agricultural chemicals, so choose organic whenever you can. It's the richest source of vitamin A, contains the most easily absorbed iron and supplies lots of vitamins B12 and D. This is a quick, easy, and healthy recipe – but not if you're pregnant as the huge amount of vitamin A could damage your baby.

Heat the oil and butter in a saucepan and sauté the onion and bacon until just turning gold. Remove with a slotted spoon and reserve. Add the liver to the pan and cook until just turning brown, about 1 minute on each side. Return the onion and bacon to the pan, pour in the sherry and heat until bubbling. Stir in the parsley and serve immediately.

mediterranean omelette flan

puff pastry	1 sheet, rolled out
garlic	3 cloves, finely chopped
tomatoes	7 ounces, seeded and roughly chopped
pitted olives	3½ ounces, rinsed and halved
mixed parsley, chervil, oregano and chives	5 tbsp freshly chopped leaves
live natural yogurt	1 cup
eggs	4

Preheat the oven to 425°F. Use the pastry to line a 9-inch deep dish pie plate. Scatter the garlic, tomatoes, and olives over the pastry and sprinkle over the herbs. Mix together the yogurt and eggs and pour over the filling. Bake in the preheated oven for 30 minutes.

large grilled shrimp on salad leaves
This recipe works excellently on a barbecue.

Pacific shrimp (or other large variety with shells)	20
garlic	5 cloves, finely chopped
extra-virgin olive oil	⅓ cup
mixed salad leaves	1 large package
lemons	2, halved

Wash the prawns under cold running water and dry thoroughly with paper towels. Mix together the garlic and olive oil in a large bowl. Add the shrimp and stir to coat thoroughly. Cover with plastic wrap and let marinate in the refrigerator for 2 hours.

Preheat the broiler to high. Remove the shrimp from the marinade with a slotted spoon and broil, basting with the marinade until the shells are almost burned, about 4 minutes on each side. Serve on a bed of salad leaves, with lemon halves to squeeze over.

dutch chicken

basmati rice	2 cups
sesame oil	3 tbsp
chicken breasts	1 pound skinless, cut into slivers along the grain
carrot	1, very thinly sliced
green bell pepper	1, seeded and very thinly sliced
Chinese five-spice powder or allspice	3 tsp
gingerroot	1¼ inches, peeled and grated
soy sauce	3 tbsp
beansprouts	8 ounces
green onions	5, trimmed and finely sliced on the diagonal

The Dutch were the first to bring Indonesian cuisine to Europe, hence the name of this recipe. In it, the combination of chicken and rice provides protein and an enormous amount of energy. The vegetables add a nutritional bonus, while the Oriental flavor of the spices makes this dish really special.

Cook the rice in a saucepan of boiling water according to the package instructions. Meanwhile, heat the oil in a preheated wok or large frying pan and stir-fry the chicken for 5 minutes. Add the carrot and green pepper and continue cooking for a further 2 minutes. Add the spices and soy sauce and stir well. Add the rest of the ingredients, including the drained rice, and cook for a further 3 minutes, still stirring vigorously.

green pasta with tuna fish

spinach tagliatelle	1 pound
extra-virgin olive oil	2 tbsp
green onions	4, large, chopped (including the green parts)
tuna	1 x 12-ounce can
tomatoes	4, large, roughly chopped

Cook the pasta in a large saucepan of boiling water according to the package instructions. Meanwhile, heat the oil in a saucepan and sauté the green onions gently until soft. Add the tuna and warm through gently. Drain the pasta and return to the pan. Mix the fish and onion mixture, with the tomatoes, into the pasta and serve.

spanish omelette

The versatility of this high-energy protein dish is that it's as good hot as it is cold. You can serve it for breakfast, lunch, or supper. The vegetables provide masses of nutrients to accompany the energy-giving potatoes.

extra-virgin olive oil	3 tbsp
new potatoes	4, small, unpeeled and cubed
red bell pepper	1, small, seeded and diced
onion	1, sliced
zucchini	2, small, diced
eggs	6
dried mixed herbs	1 tsp

Warm the olive oil in a large frying pan. Add the potatoes and stir until just turning golden. Add the pepper and onion and stir for 2 minutes until soft. Add the zucchini and stir for a further 1 minute. Beat the eggs and mix in the dried herbs. Pour the egg mixture into the pan and cook until set. Depending on how large your pan is, you may need to finish off cooking the omelette under a hot preheated broiler.

italian toast

Perfect for a Sunday morning brunch. Lots of energy from the bread, protein from the ham and cheese, plus calcium, vitamin E and all the protective nutrients in the garlic, avocado, and tomatoes.

coarse whole-wheat bread	4 thick slices
garlic	2 plump cloves, halved
extra-virgin olive oil	about 4 tbsp
avocado	1 large or 2 small, mashed just before use
tomatoes	2, large, thinly sliced
prosciutto	2 slices
mozzarella cheese	4 ounces, sliced

Preheat the broiler and line the broiler pan with foil. Toast the bread until just golden on both sides. Rub one side of each slice with the cut side of the garlic. Drizzle on a little of the olive oil. Spread the avocado on top, followed by the slices of tomato, prosciutto, and mozzarella cheese. Cook under the preheated broiler until the cheese is just melted.

gratin of potatoes and mushrooms

butter	4 tbsp
potatoes	1 pound, peeled and thinly sliced
mushrooms	8 ounces, wiped and finely sliced
salt and black pepper	to taste
basic chicken stock (see recipe, page 228)	¼ cup
light cream	¼ cup
garlic	2 cloves, very finely chopped

Preheat the oven to 350°F. Use half the butter to grease a shallow casserole. Arrange the potatoes and mushrooms in alternating layers, seasoning with salt and pepper as you go and finishing with the potatoes. Mix together the stock and cream and pour onto the dish. Dot the rest of the butter and the garlic over the top. Cover with foil and bake in the preheated oven for 1 hour. Remove the foil and leave the dish in the oven for a further 10 minutes until the potatoes are golden.

millet and mushroom risotto

extra-virgin olive oil	3 tbsp
onion	1, large, finely chopped
garlic	2 large cloves, finely chopped
millet	1 generous cup
green bell pepper	1, seeded and diced
basic chicken stock (see recipe, page 228)	3 cups
bouquet garni	1
bay leaves	2
mushrooms	8 ounces, wiped and sliced

Delicious as a brunch, this recipe combines slow-release energy from the millet, vitamin C from the pepper, and the immune-boosting properties of onions, mushrooms, and garlic.

Heat the oil in a large saucepan, add the onion and sweat until soft. Add the garlic and cook for 1 minute. Add the millet and stir for 2 minutes. Add the green pepper and cook for a further 2 minutes. Add the stock, bouquet garni, and bay leaves, cover the pan, and simmer gently for 15 minutes. Stir in the mushrooms and continue cooking for 5 minutes. Remove the bouquet garni and bay leaves before serving.

spiced chickpea casserole

canola oil	4 tbsp
onions	2, sliced
eggplant	1, sliced
bell peppers	1 red, 1 yellow, 1 green, seeded and sliced into rings
potatoes	2, large, peeled and sliced
chickpeas	1 x 14-ounce can, drained and rinsed
garlic	2 cloves, finely chopped
paprika	1 tsp
allspice	1 tsp
olive paste	2 tsp
tomato purée	2 tsp
very veggie stock (see recipe, page 227)	2 cups
chopped tomatoes	1 cup

Preheat the oven to 375°F. Heat the oil in a frying pan and sauté the onions until soft. Remove and set aside on paper towels to remove the excess oil. Using the same oil, adding more if necessary, repeat with the eggplant and peppers. Layer the vegetables and chickpeas in a casserole dish. Sprinkle over the garlic, paprika, and allspice. Mix together the olive paste, tomato purée, and 2 tbsp of water and pour over the casserole. Mix together the stock and tomatoes and pour over the dish, adding enough water to almost cover. Cover and cook in the preheated oven for 90 minutes.

posh cauliflower cheese with pasta

The pasta, oil, and cheese in this different type of traditional cauliflower cheese give you masses of energy. And as a bonus, there's the calcium in the cheese and plenty of cancer-protective nutrients in the cauliflower.

spaghetti	8 ounces
cauliflower	1, cut into small florets
extra-virgin olive oil	4 tbsp
onion	1, large, finely chopped
dry white wine	¼ cup
eggs	2, beaten
Parmesan cheese	3 tbsp, freshly grated
basil	4 tbsp roughly torn leaves

Cook the pasta according to the instructions on the package. Meanwhile, blanch the cauliflower in boiling water for 2 minutes, then drain. Heat the olive oil in a large saucepan and sauté the onion gently. Add the cauliflower and wine and simmer gently. Mix together the eggs, cheese, and half the basil. Drain the cooked pasta and add to the cauliflower. Pour over the egg mixture, stirring continuously over a gentle heat until the egg scrambles. Sprinkle over the extra basil leaves and serve.

spicy energy beans

unsalted butter	2 tbsp
onion	1, finely chopped
garlic	2 cloves, finely chopped
paprika	1 tsp
kidney beans	2 x 14-ounce cans, drained and rinsed
very veggie stock (see recipe, page 227)	2¼ cups
coriander	2 tbsp freshly chopped leaves
garam masala	1 tbsp
cooked rice	to serve

Heat the butter in a saucepan and sauté the onion gently until soft. Add the garlic and paprika. Stir thoroughly and cook over a medium heat, stirring continuously, for 2 minutes. Add the beans, stock, coriander, and garam masala. Cover and simmer for 5 minutes. Serve with rice.

steak in red wine

beef filet steaks	4, about 1 inch thick
all-purpose flour	4 tbsp
canola oil	2 tbsp
unsalted butter	2 tbsp
garlic	2 cloves, finely chopped
full-bodied red wine, such as Chianti or Barolo	1 cup
salt and black pepper	to taste

Dust the steaks with the flour. Heat the oil and butter in a large frying pan until the butter stops foaming. Add the garlic, then add the steaks and cook for 1 minute on each side. Remove the steaks and set aside. Pour in the wine and simmer, stirring continuously, until reduced by half. Season the steaks with salt and pepper, return to the pan and cook for 2–3 minutes each side, depending on how rare you like them. Serve immediately.

chillied sardine sandwiches

sardines	2 x 4-ounce cans, in olive oil
Worcestershire sauce	1 tbsp
lemon	juice of ½
whole-wheat bread	4 thick slices

Mix the sardines, including the oil, with the Worcestershire sauce and lemon. Pile the mixture onto the bread and serve.

broiled lamb chops with rosemary

lamb chops	4
extra-virgin olive oil	6 tbsp
garlic	2 cloves, finely chopped
rosemary	4 tbsp very finely chopped leaves

Trim any excess fat off the chops. Mix the oil, garlic, and rosemary together in a large shallow dish. Add the chops and turn to coat in the marinade. Cover and let marinate in the refrigerator for 2 hours, turning occasionally.

Preheat the broiler to high. Remove the chops from the marinade, leaving some of the liquid still clinging, and broil for 2–3 minutes on each side. Serve immediately.

brown rice risotto with sun-dried tomatoes

Strictly speaking, you cook risotto by stirring the stock in gradually over about 30 minutes. But this dish is more of a boiled rice with vegetables than a risotto. It's easier, extremely high in energy, and delicious hot or cold.

canola oil	3 tbsp
onion	1, finely chopped
garlic	2 cloves, finely chopped
brown rice	1⅓ cups
sun-dried tomatoes	8 ounces
tomatoes	4, roughly chopped
very veggie stock (see recipe, page 227)	3 cups
Cheddar cheese	3 tbsp, grated
basil	10 leaves, roughly torn

Heat the oil in a large non-stick frying pan and sauté the onion and garlic gently until just turning golden. Add the rice, sun-dried tomatoes snipped to the size of a raisin, fresh tomatoes, and stock. Simmer for 40 minutes, adding extra stock or water, if necessary. Stir in the cheese, sprinkle on the basil, and serve.

unsalted butter	4 tbsp
duck breasts	4, skinless
onion	1, finely chopped
green peppercorns	2 tbsp
red wine	⅓ cup
sour cream	4 tbsp

duck breasts with pepper sauce

Heat the butter in a large frying pan and sauté the duck breasts for about 4 minutes until they are golden. Remove and keep warm. Add the onion to the pan and sauté until golden. Add the peppercorns and red wine and simmer for 10 minutes. Add the crème fraîche and continue to simmer for 3 minutes. Meanwhile, slice the duck breasts diagonally and arrange on the serving plates. Pour over the peppercorn sauce and serve.

zucchini	4, small, halved lengthwise
eggplant	1, large, sliced widthwise
bell peppers	1 red, 1 yellow, seeded and cut into wide strips
extra-virgin olive oil	5 tbsp
Little Gem lettuces	2, broken into leaves
portobello mushroom	1, large, wiped and quartered
garlic	2 cloves, finely chopped
mozzarella cheese	2 ounces, sliced

broiled italian vegetables

Preheat the broiler and line the broiler pan with foil. Add the vegetables and brush with half the olive oil. Cook for 3 minutes on each side. Put the lettuce onto an ovenproof plate and place the mushroom quarters on top. Arrange the grilled vegetables over the whole dish, then drizzle over the rest of the oil and sprinkle over the garlic. Top with the mozzarella slices and return to the hot broiler for 1 minute or until the cheese has melted.

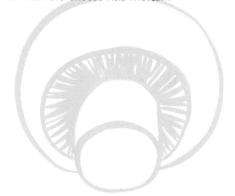

sage	16 leaves
sunflower oil	4 tbsp
unsalted butter	4 tbsp
calves' liver	8 thin slices, weighing about 1 pound in total
limes	2, halved, to serve

roman liver

Fry the sage leaves in the oil for 1 minute until crisp. Remove with a slotted spoon and drain on paper towels. Wipe the pan and add the butter. Heat until foaming, add the liver slices and cook for 1 minute on each side. Serve with the sage leaves on top and the lime halves on the side.

shrimp and tomato curry

onion	1, very finely chopped
tomatoes	1 x 14-ounce can
garlic	1 clove, very finely chopped
coriander	4 tbsp freshly chopped leaves
frozen peas	¼ cup
very veggie stock (see recipe, page 227)	¾ cup
ground coriander	1 tsp
ground cumin	1 tsp
sun-dried tomato paste	2 tbsp
curry powder	1 tsp
red chile	1, seeded and very finely chopped
cooked peeled shrimp	1 pound
sour cream	1 x 8-ounce tub
cooked rice	to serve

This is a variation on traditional kedgeree. It overflows with a combination of protective nutrients which will boost and enhance your radiance.

Put the onion, tomatoes, garlic, half the fresh coriander, the peas and the stock in a large saucepan and simmer for 5 minutes. Mix together the ground coriander, cumin, tomato paste, curry powder and chile. Add to the stock and simmer for a further 5 minutes. Add the shrimp and simmer for 3 minutes. Sprinkle with the remaining fresh coriander, stir in the sour cream and serve on a bed of rice.

potted shrimp

unsalted butter	12 tbsp
allspice	2 tsp
lemon	juice of ½
shrimp	1 pound, 5 ounces peeled weight, thoroughly thawed if bought frozen
bay leaves	3

Melt the butter in a medium saucepan. Add the allspice and lemon juice and let stand, off the heat, for 10 minutes. Put the shrimp into a shallow 3-cup dish. Strain the butter over them, pushing them down so that all the shrimp are covered. Push in the bay leaves, making sure they're covered by the butter, too. Cover and let cool in the refrigerator until the butter solidifies – at least 1 hour.

stir-fried turkey breast with vegetables and noodles

egg noodles	1 pound
canola oil	2 tbsp
gingerroot	1 inch, grated
garlic	10 cloves, peeled
red chile	1, seeded and finely chopped
turkey breast	1 pound, fincly cubed
onion	1, small, finely chopped
mixed vegetables – baby carrots, broccoli, snow peas, corn, cauliflower, cabbage, or a package of stir-fry vegetables	1 pound, finely chopped
sesame oil	2 tbsp
soy sauce	1 tbsp

Turkey is a good source of protein and essential B vitamins, but is virtually fat-free. Mixed here with the skin-nourishing root vegetables and circulation-stimulating ginger and chile, this is an all-year-round radiance-enhancing recipe.

Cook the noodles according to the package instructions. Meanwhile, heat the oil in a preheated wok or large saucepan and stir-fry the ginger, garlic, chile, and turkey for 2 minutes. Add the onion and vegetables and stir in the sesame oil. Stir-fry for a further 4 minutes, adding the soy sauce gradually, until the vegetables are just beginning to crisp. Remove from the heat. Drain the cooked noodles, mix into the stir-fry, and serve immediately.

non-meatballs in tomato sauce

vegeburger mix	1 pound
garlic	3 cloves, finely chopped
mint	2 tbsp freshly chopped leaves
parsley	2 tbsp freshly chopped leaves
tomatoes	1 x 14-ounce can
vegetable stock cube	1
white wine	4 tbsp
onion	1, large, finely chopped
extra-virgin olive oil	1 tbsp
green chile	1, seeded and finely chopped
canola oil	⅓ cup

Prepare the vegeburger mix according to the package instructions, adding the garlic, mint, and parsley. Put the tomatoes and their juice into a large frying pan with the crumbled stock cube, wine, onion, olive oil, and chile. Bring to the boil and simmer for 10 minutes. While the sauce is cooking, form the vegeburger mixture into walnut-sized balls and fry gently in the canola oil for 3 minutes on each side. Add them to the tomato sauce and serve immediately.

eggs florentine

baby spinach	2 pounds
unsalted butter	4 tbsp
all-purpose flour	3 tbsp
2 percent milk	½ cup
tarragon	4 large sprigs, leaves removed and chopped
eggs	4, large

Preheat the oven to 325°F. Wash the spinach, even if the packet says it's already washed. Put into a saucepan with just the water clinging to it. Add half the butter, cover the pan, and cook over a low heat until wilted, about 5 minutes. Divide between 4 medium ramekin dishes.

Heat the remaining butter in a small saucepan, add the flour and milk and cook gently until you have a roux. Reduce the heat to minimum, add the tarragon, and simmer for 3 minutes. Put half the mixture into the ramekins. Crack an egg into each. Top with the rest of the tarragon sauce and bake in the preheated oven for 20 minutes.

salmon fishcakes with tomato salsa

crushed tomatoes	2 x 14-ounce cans
garlic	4 cloves, finely chopped
red chiles	2, seeded and finely chopped
capers	2 tbsp, rinsed
canola oil	⅓ cup
onion	1, finely chopped
salmon	1 x 7.5-ounce can, drained
whole-wheat breadcrumbs	6 tbsp
dill	2 tbsp freshly chopped leaves
parsley	2 tbsp freshly chopped leaves
eggs	2, beaten

Make the tomato salsa by putting the first 4 ingredients in a blender and whizzing until smooth. Set aside until required.

Heat 2 tbsp of the oil in a saucepan and sauté the onion gently until golden, about 5 minutes. Meanwhile, put the fish in a bowl and mash with a fork. Mix with the breadcrumbs, dill, and parsley and mix in the eggs. Using your hands, make into tangerine-size mounds and flatten to about ½ inch thick. Heat the remaining oil in a frying pan and fry the cakes for 3 minutes on each side until golden. Serve with the salsa.

potato cake with broccoli

potatoes	2 pounds, peeled and grated
eggs	2
broccoli	5 ounces, cut into small florets
onion	1, finely chopped
parsley	3 tbsp finely chopped leaves
garlic	2 cloves, finely chopped
canola oil	5 tbsp
all-purpose flour	2 tbsp

In this posh form of bubble and squeak, it's the broccoli that adds the super-radiant nutrients. This is a great way to encourage acne-prone adolescents to eat their greens.

Mix together the potatoes, eggs, broccoli, onion, parsley, and garlic. Heat the oil in a large frying pan and add the potato mixture, flatten with a fork and sprinkle the flour on top. Cook over a medium heat until the bottom is golden, about 10 minutes. Preheat the broiler to hot and transfer the frying pan underneath it. Broil until the top is golden. Slide the potato cake onto paper towels to soak up any excess oil, then onto a plate to serve.

broiled sole with cheese

sole fillets	4
salt and black pepper	to season
unsalted butter	4 tbsp
Dijon mustard	4 tsp
Cheddar cheese	4 tbsp, grated

Season the fillets with salt and pepper. Preheat the broiler to its highest setting and line the broiler pan with foil. Brush the foil with the butter, then put the fillets on top. Put under the broiler for 1 minute and then turn. Brush with the mustard, sprinkle on the cheese and return to the broiler until the fish is cooked, about 3 minutes.

quick chickpea hot pot

olive oil	4 tbsp
onion	1, finely chopped
garlic	3 cloves, finely chopped
tomatoes	1 x 14-ounce can
chickpeas	1 x 14-ounce can
frozen mixed vegetables	1 pound
bouquet garni	1 sachet
stock	3½ cups
parsley	2 tbsp freshly chopped leaves

Cheap, filling, easy to use but much ignored, chickpeas are an excellent radiance food. Apart from their cleansing fiber and B vitamins, they also contain minerals essential for maintaining the structure and elasticity of the skin.

Heat the olive oil in a large saucepan and sauté the onion and garlic gently until just soft. Pour in the tomatoes with their juice and bring to a simmer. Meanwhile, drain and rinse the chickpeas. Add the chickpeas, mixed vegetables, bouquet garni sachet and stock to the onion and garlic mixture and simmer for 15 minutes. Sprinkle with the chopped parsley and serve.

lentil and barley pilaf

pearl barley	⅔ cup
very veggie stock	2¼ cups
(see recipe, page 227)	
brown lentils	1⅓ cups
olive oil	4 tbsp
carrot	1, finely chopped
celery	1 stalk, finely chopped
onions	2, sliced into rings
parsley	1 tbsp freshly chopped leaves
live natural yogurt	¾ cup

Wash the barley, soak in cold water to cover for 1 hour and drain. Put the stock into a large saucepan, add the barley and simmer, covered, for 45 minutes or until tender. Meanwhile, cook the lentils according to the package instructions (this normally takes 30–40 minutes). Heat 1 tbsp of the oil in a frying pan and sauté the carrot, celery, and half the onions gently for 4 minutes. Mix with the barley and lentils and keep warm in a 350°F oven. Heat the rest of the oil in a frying pan and fry the remaining onion. Serve the pilaf garnished with the onion rings and parsley and with the yogurt on the side.

chicken liver kebabs

wooden skewers	4
chicken livers	8 ounces
unsalted butter	8 tbsp
shallots	4, very finely chopped
sage	12 leaves
cremini mushrooms	8, stems removed
cherry tomatoes	12, halved
red bell pepper	1, seeded and cubed

Another recipe for outer and inner radiance. The chicken livers are full of iron and B vitamins for healthy blood, there's lycopene in the tomatoes, betacarotene and vitamin C in the peppers, and the bonus of mind-boosting essential oils in the sage.

Soak the skewers in water for 30 minutes before using to prevent burning. Preheat the broiler and line the broiler rack with foil. Wash and dry the chicken livers, cutting off any membranes. Heat half the butter in a saucepan and sauté the chicken livers and shallots for 2 minutes, stirring continuously. Remove with a slotted spoon and keep warm. Add the sage leaves to the pan and sauté until slightly crisp. Remove and keep warm. Thread the chicken livers onto the kebab sticks, alternating them with the remaining ingredients. Brush each kebab with the remaining butter and broil for 5 minutes, turning once. Alternatively, cook on a barbecue.

stuffed green bell peppers

green lentils, preferably Puy	1¾ cups, washed
green bell peppers	4, large
extra-virgin olive oil	4 tbsp
onions	2, finely chopped
garlic	3 cloves, finely chopped
Worcestershire sauce	2 tbsp
Cheddar cheese	8 ounces, grated

Preheat the oven to 350°F. Cook the lentils according to the package instructions (this normally takes 30–40 minutes). Meanwhile, halve the peppers widthwise, seed and put into a large baking pan, add 1 inch of water and bake in the preheated oven for 40 minutes.

Heat the oil in a saucepan and sauté the onion and garlic until soft. Drain the lentils, reserving 4 tbsp of their cooking liquid, and mix this liquid together with the lentils and Worcestershire sauce into the onion and garlic. Pile the mixture into the peppers. Sprinkle with the cheese and return to the oven for 15 minutes.

zucchini pasta

thin pasta, such as spaghettini	1 pound
zucchini	4, grated
gingerroot	2 inches, grated
light soy sauce	2 tbsp
extra-virgin olive oil	4 tsp
Parmesan cheese	4 tsp, freshly grated
green onions	4, finely chopped
beansprouts	4 ounces

Cook the pasta in a saucepan of boiling water according to the package instructions. Transfer to a large serving bowl and mix in all the other ingredients. Serve immediately.

pasta with tuna fish and black olives

Quicker than take-out, the olives and their oil in this 15-minute recipe provide plenty of skin-nourishing vitamin E and mono-unsaturated fat, while the fish contains anti-inflammatory essential acids. In addition, there's an energy boost from the pasta.

tomatoes	1 x 14-ounce can
vegetable stock cube	1
white wine	2 tbsp
onion	1, very finely chopped
olive oil	2 tbsp
red or green chile	1, seeded and finely chopped
mixed parsley, basil and coriander	1 tbsp, freshly chopped leaves
tuna	1 x 6-ounce can, in oil, drained and flaked
black olives	10, pitted
pasta	8 ounces

Put the tomatoes, with their juice, into a large saucepan. Add the crumbled stock cube, wine, onion, olive oil, and chile. Simmer for 10 minutes and add the herbs. Mix in the tuna and olives. Heat through gently while you cook the pasta in a large saucepan according to the packet instructions. Stir the sauce into the pasta and serve.

tofu, vegetable, and cashew nut stir-fry

This is the ultimate radiance meal, with natural plant hormones from the tofu, antibacterial sulphur from the cabbage, masses of vitamin A from the carrots, and more than your day's requirement of vitamin C.

olive oil	3 tbsp
tofu	8 ounces, drained and cubed
onion	1, finely chopped
green bell pepper	1, seeded and cubed
gingerroot	½ inch, grated
celery	1 stalk, finely sliced
carrots	2, finely sliced
cabbage	½, shredded
mushrooms	4 ounces, wiped and sliced
cashew nuts	4 ounces
very veggie stock (see recipe, page 227)	8 ounces
soy sauce	1 tsp

Heat the oil in a preheated wok, add the tofu, and fry gently until golden brown. Remove from the wok with a slotted spoon and reserve. Add the onion, green pepper, ginger, and celery and sauté gently until soft. Add the carrots and cabbage and sauté for 4 minutes. Add the mushrooms and cashew nuts and cook for a further 1 minute. Pour in the stock, cover, and simmer until the vegetables are soft. Just before serving, add the fried tofu and the soy sauce.

bean stew or hot pot

olive oil	1 tsp
onion	1, finely chopped
garlic	2 cloves, finely chopped
chili powder	1 tbsp
mustard powder	1 large pinch
white wine vinegar	2 tbsp
tomato purée	1 tbsp
Worcestershire sauce	1 tsp
crushed tomatoes	1 cup
very veggie stock (see recipe, page 227)	2 cups
mixed root vegetables – carrots, rutabagas, parsnips, turnips etc	2 pounds, diced
mushrooms	4 ounces, sliced
chickpeas	1 cup, cooked
borlotti beans	1 cup, cooked

The beans in this delicious casserole are a source of natural plant hormones, which give a brilliant radiance boost. With the betacarotene and minerals from the root vegetables and masses of cancer-protective and skin-nourishing lycopene from the tomatoes, this is a wonderful meal for chilly autumn or winter evenings. And the leftovers are even nicer heated up the following day.

Heat the oil in a large saucepan and sauté the onion and garlic until soft. Add the chili powder, mustard, and vinegar and simmer for 1 minute. Mix in the tomato purée, Worcestershire sauce, tomatoes, and stock. Add the root vegetables and simmer for 20 minutes until tender. Add the mushrooms, drained and rinsed chickpeas, and beans, and cook for a further 5 minutes.

creamy mackerel with eggs

smoked mackerel fillets	8 ounces, flaked
light cream	3 tbsp
lemon	juice of ½
green onions	4, large, finely chopped
butter	4 tbsp
eggs	6
parsley	2 tbsp finely chopped leaves
whole wheat toast	to serve

This sounds like a strange mixture, but it makes a delicious weekend brunch, breakfast, or light supper. Smoked mackerel contains less salt than smoked salmon, has a fuller flavor and all the health benefits of oily fish.

Mix the mackerel fillets with the cream, lemon juice, and green onions In a large bowl. Set aside. Heat the butter in a nonstick frying pan. Add the eggs and gently break up the yolks. Continue cooking, pushing the egg mixture in toward the center of the pan – you want the yolks and whites to stay slightly separate. When the eggs are beginning to set, add the mackerel mixture and stir until you have the consistency you prefer. Scatter with the parsley and serve immediately with whole-wheat toast.

baked halibut with mushrooms

unsalted butter	about 4 tbsp
halibut steaks	4
shallots or small onions	3, very finely chopped
oyster mushrooms	5 ounces, wiped and sliced
dry white wine	½ cup
lemon	juice of ½
parsley	2 tbsp freshly chopped leaves

Preheat the oven to 375°F. Rub half the butter over the base of a large, shallow ovenproof dish and put the halibut in it. Melt the rest of the butter and sauté the shallots and mushrooms gently until soft. Cover the fish with the shallots and mushrooms, pour over the wine and bake in the preheated oven for 20–25 minutes. Sprinkle over the lemon juice and parsley and serve.

chicken with thyme and lemon

whole-wheat flour	3 tbsp
dried thyme	2 tsp
chicken thighs	8
milk	½ cup
canola oil	4 tbsp
lemon	juice of 1

Preheat the oven to 375°F. Mix the flour and thyme together in a large bowl. Dip the chicken in the milk and roll in the flour mixture. Heat the oil in large frying pan and fry the chicken until browned on all sides. Transfer the chicken to a wire rack placed over a roasting pan and pour over the lemon juice. Bake in the preheated oven for 15 minutes.

pita bread pizza

whole-wheat pitas	4
tomatoes	4, sliced
dried oregano	1 tsp
Cheddar cheese	4 tbsp, grated
extra-virgin olive oil	4 tsp

Preheat the broiler to high and toast the pitas on one side for 1 minute. Turn them over, arrange the tomatoes on top, sprinkle with the oregano, then the cheese. Drizzle the oil on top and return to the broiler until the cheese is bubbling, about 2 minutes.

risotto con salsa cruda

This rice and raw vegetable dish provides nutrients at their best. None of the essential ingredients is lost in cooking, which means you get optimum radiance benefits with minimum effort.

Put the vegetables in a bowl, mix in the oil and let marinate for half an hour. Meanwhile, cook the rice according to the package instructions. Remove from the heat and leave uncovered for 10 minutes to dry and separate. Drain if necessary. While the rice is still warm, mix it into the mixed vegetables and sprinkle on the herbs.

cucumber	1, peeled, seeded and finely cubed
tomatoes	4, coarsely chopped
green onions	4, finely sliced
garlic	2 cloves, finely chopped
carrots	4, very finely cubed
radishes	4, halved
zucchini	3, small, finely cubed
fresh peas	⅓ cup
extra-virgin olive oil	4 tbsp
long-grain brown rice	1½ cups
chives	1 tbsp, snipped
parsley	1 tbsp freshly chopped leaves

grilled paprika chicken

Mix the paprika, pepper, lemon, oil, and garlic together in a bowl. Put the chicken breasts in a large, shallow dish and pour over the marinade. Cover and refrigerate for at least 1 hour.

Preheat the broiler and line the broiler pan with foil. Remove the chicken from the marinade and place on the broiler rack. Broil for 6–7 minutes on each side, depending on thickness, basting occasionally with the marinade.

paprika	1 tsp
freshly ground black pepper	2 good grindings
lemon	juice and grated rind of 1
canola oil	4 tbsp
garlic	2 cloves, very finely chopped
chicken breasts	4, skinless and boneless, flattened

griddled tuna with roasted vegetables and fusilli

extra-virgin olive oil	⅓ cup
rosemary	1 large sprig
garlic	2 cloves, finely chopped
tuna steaks	4
canola oil	⅓ cup
bell peppers	1 red, 1 green, seeded and cut into thick strips
onions	2, quartered
zucchini	4, small, halved lengthwise
fennel	1 bulb, quartered lengthwise
baby leeks	2, halved lengthwise
fusilli	1 pound

Fresh tuna is an excellent source of radiant-boosting essential fatty acids, and the fennel, with its hint of licorice flavor, helps to stimulate the cleansing functions of the liver. This is a versatile dish that you can also cook under a hot broiler or on a summer barbecue.

Put the olive oil, rosemary, and garlic into a large, shallow dish. Add the tuna and coat in the mixture. Cover and refrigerate. Meanwhile, preheat the oven to 425°F. Put the canola oil into a baking dish, add the vegetables and stir to coat well. Roast in the preheated oven for 30 minutes, stirring occasionally. When the vegetables are nearly ready, cook the fusilli in a large saucepan of boiling water according to the package instructions.

Preheat a griddle pan. Remove the tuna from the marinade, leaving some of the oil still clinging, and cook in the griddle pan over a high heat for 2 minutes on each side. Serve in a mound, with the fusilli on the bottom, then the vegetables and the tuna on top.

sage burgers

mixed nuts	8 ounces
whole-wheat breadcrumbs	¾ cup
sunflower oil	about 4 tbsp
onion	1, very finely chopped
very veggie stock (see recipe, page 227)	1 cup
marmite or vegemite	2 tsp
sage	6 leaves, finely chopped
whole-wheat flour	4 tbsp

These are a highly nutritious alternative to meat-based burgers, with the bonus that they contain no saturated fat. Added to that, they are rich in skin-friendly minerals, especially zinc and selenium, and have lots of fiber, which encourages good digestion. The nuts also provide radiance-enhancing vitamin E.

Grind the nuts and breadcrumbs in a food processor or blender. Heat 2 tbsp of the oil in a saucepan and sauté the onion gently until soft. Heat the stock and marmite together in a separate saucepan until blended. Mix the ground nuts and breadcrumbs with the onion, adding enough of the stock and marmite mixture to make a good consistency. Shape into 4 burgers and dust with the flour. Heat the rest of the oil in a large frying pan and shallow-fry the burgers for 4 minutes on each side.

lamb and pine-nut koftas

wooden skewers	4
onion	1, coarsely chopped
pine nuts	¼ cup
ground lamb	1 pound, fresh
mint	2 tbsp freshly chopped leaves
egg	1
pita bread	to serve
green salad	to serve

Soak the skewers in water for 30 minutes before using to prevent burning. Preheat the broiler and line the broiler rack with foil. Put the onion and pine nuts into a food processor or blender and chop finely. Add the lamb, mint, and egg and blend to a smoothish purée. Mold into walnut-sized balls and thread onto skewers. Broil for 2 minutes on each side. Serve with pita bread and a green salad.

one-pot pasta with vegetables and pesto

spaghetti	1 pound
green beans	2½ ounces, finely chopped
zucchini	2, finely diced
new potatoes	3, very finely diced
pesto sauce	4 tbsp
Parmesan cheese	3 tbsp, freshly grated

Another quick, easy, and inexpensive meal with minimum effort and maximum benefit. As well as the skin-friendly nutrients in the vegetables, there's added value from the mood-enhancing essential oils in basil.

Bring a large saucepan of water to the boil and add the spaghetti and vegetables. They will all be just tender at the same time, about 6 minutes. Drain, reserving 2 tsp of the water and mix this in a bowl with the pesto. Mix the pesto with the drained pasta and vegetables. Add the Parmesan and serve immediately.

beef and ginger stir-fry

cornstarch	1 tbsp
Chinese five-spice powder	½ tsp
soy sauce	3 tbsp
lean grilling steak – fillet is best	1 pound, cut into thin strips
sesame oil	3 tbsp
gingerroot	1 inch, grated
garlic	2 cloves, very finely chopped
red bell epper	1, small, seeded and finely cubed
broccoli	1 head, florets separated and stalks finely sliced
green onions	4, sliced diagonally
sherry	½ cup
cooked rice or noodles	to serve

Mix the cornstarch, Chinese five-spice powder, and soy sauce together in a large bowl. Add the steak and stir to coat thoroughly. Cover and let marinate in the refrigerator for about 20 minutes. Heat the oil in a preheated wok or large frying pan and add the steak, ginger, and garlic. Stir-fry for 4 minutes. Add the pepper, broccoli florets and stalks, and green onions, and continue cooking for a further 2 minutes. Pour in the sherry, cover the pan, and cook for 1 minute. Serve with rice or noodles.

ten-minute mussels

unsalted butter	4 tbsp
shallots	4, very finely chopped
garlic	very finely chopped
red chile	1, seeded and finely chopped
parsley	5 tbsp freshly chopped leaves
dry white wine	½ bottle
mussels	4 pounds, washed, beards removed and any open shells discarded

Melt the butter in a pan large enough to hold all the mussels and sauté the shallots, garlic, and chile gently. Add the chopped parsley, pour in the wine, and bring to the boil. Add the mussels. Cover the pan and cook over a medium heat for 5 minutes until the shells open. Discard any that don't open. Using a slotted spoon, put the mussels into serving bowls. Bring the rest of the liquid to a very fast boil for 3 minutes. Pour over the mussels and serve.

squash, almond, and raisin bulgur

bulgur	1 cup
olive oil	at least 6 tbsp
onions	2, large, very finely sliced
squash or zucchini	12 ounces, peeled, seeded and cubed
ground coriander	1-2 tsp
ground cumin	1-2 tsp
sliced almonds	⅔ cup
raisins	⅔ cup
salt and black pepper	to taste

This energy-giving vegetable dish is another fast/slow energy meal thanks to the fruit, the sugar, and the grains. If you've never cooked with bulgur before, do try this recipe. It's a wonderful wheat and cooking it is as easy as cooking rice.

Simmer the bulgur in twice its volume of water for 10 minutes until most of the water is absorbed. Meanwhile, heat 2 tbsp of the oil and fry the onion until it is brown but not crisp. Add the squash and sauté until brown, adding more oil if necessary. Sprinkle in the spices and cook for 1 minute, stirring continuously. Reduce the heat, add the almonds and raisins, and continue cooking, still stirring, until the almonds are golden. Drain the bulgur, if necessary, and stir into the vegetable mixture. Season to taste with salt and black pepper. Add more oil if the mixture looks too dry and heat through for 1 minute.

braised chicken

canola oil	4 tbsp
shallots	8, halved
smoked bacon	4 strips, snipped into 6 pieces each
chicken	1, weighing about 3 pounds
mushrooms	6 ounces, sliced
white wine	½ cup
bouquet garni	1 sachet
bay leaves	2
new potatoes	1 pound, small

Preheat the oven to 375°F. Heat the oil in a metal casserole dish large enough to hold the chicken. Sauté the shallots and bacon for 4 minutes, then remove from the dish and reserve. Add the chicken and brown on all sides. Return the onion and bacon to the dish, along with the mushrooms, wine, bouquet garni, and bay leaves. Cover and bake in the preheated oven for 45 minutes. Add the potatoes and continue baking for a further 30 minutes. Remove the bouquet garni and bay leaves before serving.

stuffed red bell peppers

red bell peppers	2, with flat bottoms, halved widthwise and seeded
extra-virgin olive oil	4 tbsp
onion	1, finely chopped
garlic	2 cloves, finely chopped
pine nuts	2 tbsp
spinach	8 ounces
basmati rice	⅔ cup, cooked
Parmesan cheese	4 tbsp, freshly grated

Preheat the oven to 350°F. Put the peppers in a lightly greased baking pan. Heat the oil in a small saucepan and add the onion and garlic. Cook until the onion is soft. Add the pine nuts and continue cooking until the pine nuts are just golden.

Meanwhile, wash the spinach and put into a saucepan with just the water clinging to it. Cover and simmer gently until just wilted. Mix together the rice, garlic, onions, pine nuts, and spinach. Pile the mixture into the 4 pepper halves, cover lightly with foil, and bake in the preheated oven for 30 minutes. Remove the foil. Top with the Parmesan cheese and return to the oven for a further 10 minutes. Serve.

soups and salads

If you're taking the trouble and making the effort to detox, you're serious about your health. So you won't mind the extra work involved in making your own stock and good salad dressings – the rewards in terms of health-giving nutrients and absence of salt and unwanted chemicals far outweigh the effort.

very veggie stock

onions	2 – 1 peeled and quartered, 1 left whole
celery	3 large stalks, with their leaves
leek	1
parsnip	1
sage	1 large sprig
thyme	2 sprigs
bay leaves	6
parsley	2 generous handfuls
black peppercorns	12, whole
water	2 quarts

This basic recipe may seem as if it takes a long time and will leave you with far more stock that you need. But it's simple to make and healthier than any commercial stock or cube. If you don't need all of it, you can boil it down until it has reduced to half its volume, put it into the freezer – I often freeze it in ice-cube trays – then add it to an equal amount of boiling water and use as required.

Put all the ingredients into a large saucepan, cutting them to fit if necessary. Bring slowly to the boil and simmer for 40 minutes. Strain and use as needed.

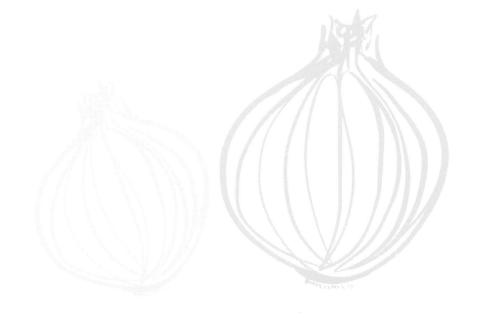

basic chicken stock

chicken	1 carcass – the remains of a roast chicken will do, but it's better to ask a butcher to keep a carcass that has been stripped of its other useful meat
water	2 quarts
green onions	6, with the stems on
leek	1, large, cleaned, trimmed and coarsely chopped
celery	2 large stalks, chopped
rosemary	1 large sprig
parsley	2 generous handfuls
sage	1 large sprig
thyme	2 large sprigs
bay leaves	3
white peppercorns	10

Put the chicken carcass into a large heavy-based saucepan and cover with the water. Bring to the boil and cook, uncovered, for 30 minutes. Add the rest of the ingredients, partially cover the pan and simmer for 40 minutes, adding more water if necessary. Strain and use as needed.

traditional chicken soup

chicken	1 carcass
water	5 cups
bouquet garni	1 sachet
bay leaves	3
new potatoes	8 ounces
mixed carrots, parsnips, turnips and rutabaga	1 pound, cut into even-sized cubes
leeks	2, cleaned, trimmed and thickly sliced
celery	2 stalks, thickly sliced
Parmesan cheese	4 tbsp, freshly grated

Jewish penicillin may be a joke, but scientific evidence now proves that it really does work. With all the root vegetables, this is a great energy-giver too.

Put the chicken carcass in a large saucepan and pour over the water. Add the bouquet garni and bay leaves and simmer for about 1 hour. Remove the carcass from the pan and fork off any loosened meat. Halve or quarter the potatoes if large, then add with the rest of the vegetables and simmer until tender, about 30 minutes. Remove and discard the bouquet garni and bay leaves. Ladle into soup bowls and serve sprinkled with the Parmesan cheese.

lettuce soup

Perfect as an evening snack as lettuce helps you sleep, and it's a great way to use up a glut of garden lettuces.
Heat the oil and sauté the onion gently for 2 minutes. Add the garlic and continue cooking for a further 1 minute. Add the shredded lettuce and stir until wilted. Pour in the stock, then add the tarragon and simmer for 5 minutes. Serve with spoonfuls of sour cream floating on top.

extra-virgin olive oil	4 tbsp
sweet onion	1, large, very finely chopped
garlic	2 cloves, very finely chopped
Little Gem lettuce	2 heads, shredded
very veggie stock (see recipe, page 227)	1 quart
tarragon	4 large sprigs, leaves freshly chopped
sour cream	½ cup

vegetable soup

One bowl gives at least three portions of health-boosting vegetables.
Heat the oil and sauté the onion and garlic for 5 minutes. Add the carrots, leeks, and zucchini and continue cooking for a further 5 minutes. Pour in the stock and tomato purée and simmer until the vegetables are soft. Add the parsley and peas and continue cooking for about 5 minutes.

onion	1, large, peeled and finely chopped
garlic	2 cloves, finely chopped
carrots	2, large, diced
leeks	3, cleaned, trimmed, and sliced
zucchini	4, peeled and thinly sliced
very veggie stock (see recipe, page 227)	3 cups
tomato purée	3 tbsp
parsley	1 large bunch, leaves finely chopped
fresh or frozen peas	⅔ cup

chicken soup with barley

The ultimate healing soup, this is a one-pot meal providing protein, carbohydrates, vitamins, minerals, and trace elements.

extra-virgin olive oil	4 tbsp
onion	1, large, finely chopped
carrot	1, large, finely sliced
leek	1, large, white part only, finely sliced
basic chicken stock (see recipe, page 228)	3½ cups
pearl barley	2 tbsp, washed
bay leaves	4
peppercorns	6, black
chicken carcass	1, skin removed
fresh or frozen peas	¼ cup
fresh or frozen fava beans	¼ cup

Heat the oil in a saucepan and sauté the onion, carrot, and leek gently for 5 minutes. Add the stock, barley, bay leaves, peppercorns, and chicken carcass. Cover and simmer for 2 hours, skimming away any scum that rises to the surface with a slotted spoon.

Remove the pan from the heat and let cool. Lift out the chicken carcass, remove any meat from it and return this to the pan. Remove and discard the bay leaves. Add the peas and beans. Return the pan to the heat and simmer for 7 minutes.

borscht

This traditional Eastern European soup is excellent for general health, but especially valuable if you have anemia, chronic fatigue, or tired-all-the-time syndrome.

canola oil	2 tbsp
onion	1, peeled and finely sliced
garlic	2 cloves, finely chopped
fennel	1 large bulb, finely chopped
beets	1 pound, raw, peeled and finely sliced
carrot	1, large, peeled and sliced
very veggie stock (see recipe, page 227)	1 quart
thyme	1 large sprig
rosemary	1 large sprig
bay leaves	4
lemon	juice of 1
live natural yogurt	4 ounces, to serve

Heat the oil gently in a large saucepan and sauté the onion, garlic, fennel, beet, and carrot for about 10 minutes. Pour in the stock and herbs and simmer for about 30 minutes until the vegetables are soft.

Remove and discard the herbs. Transfer the remaining ingredients to a blender or food processor and whiz until smooth. Stir in the lemon juice. Serve with a swirl of yogurt in each bowl.

thick bean and barley soup

The combination of cereal and legumes provides an abundance of protein, but the bonus comes from the plant hormones in the beans. Perfect for all menstrual problems and ideal for older women as it helps prevent bone loss – great for men, too.

pearl barley	2 tbsp
very veggie stock (see recipe, page 227)	1 quart
carrots	3, peeled and cubed
turnip	1, large, peeled and cubed
parsnip	1, peeled and cubed
celery	2 stalks, with leaves, finely sliced
tomato purée	2 large tbsp
mixed chervil, parsley, oregano, marjoram, and sage	4 large tbsp, finely chopped
borlotti, black-eye peas, red kidney, white, flageolet or other beans	1 cup cooked or canned, drained
parsley	2 tbsp freshly chopped leaves, to garnish

Put the barley and stock in a large saucepan and simmer for about 40 minutes until the barley is soft. Add the vegetables, tomato purée, and herbs. Bring back to the boil and simmer for a further 15 minutes. Add the beans and continue to simmer for another 15 minutes, until the beans are soft. Serve with the extra parsley scattered on top.

white soup

The best soup in the world to protect your heart.

ground almonds	1½ cups
garlic	2 cloves, very finely chopped
white organic bread	2 thick slices, soaked in water and squeezed dry
extra-virgin olive oil	
ice water	about 3 cups
lemon juice	2 tbsp
seedless white grapes	20, halved

Put the almonds, garlic and bread in a food processor and whiz until smooth. With the machine running, gradually add the olive oil until the mixture is the consistency of mayonnaise. Pour in the ice water until you have the texture of heavy cream. Stir in the lemon juice. Serve with the grapes floating on top.

cold beet and apple soup

beets	1 pound, raw, peeled and grated
onion	1, finely sliced
apple juice	1 quart
lemon	juice of 1
sour cream	¾ cup
salt and black pepper	to taste

Beets have a natural high sugar content, making them an excellent source of energy. They also have significant blood-building properties and are extremely rich in betacarotene, which your body converts into vitamin A – one of the most important of all the radiance nutrients. Here beets are combined with health-giving apples to create an unusual soup that is refreshing for those hot, exhausting summer days.

Put the beets and onion into a food processor or blender with half the apple juice and whiz until smooth. Add the rest of the juice, plus the lemon juice and sour cream. Stir well, season to taste with salt and pepper and chill in the refrigerator until ready to serve.

cabbage soup with potatoes

carrots	2, large
Savoy cabbage	¼, roughly chopped
potatoes	12 ounces, peeled and cubed
onion	1, large, finely sliced
very veggie stock (see recipe, page 227)	5 cups
chives	20 stems
dill	3 sprigs
freshly ground nutmeg	2 pinches

Trim the carrots, peel if not organic, and slice. Put the cabbage, potatoes, onion, and carrots into a large saucepan. Add the stock and simmer until the potatoes and carrots are tender. Add the chives, dill, and nutmeg. Transfer the soup to a blender or food processor and whiz until smooth. Alternatively, use an immersion blender. Ladle into soup bowls and serve.

hauser broth

carrots	4 ounces
celery	3 stalks, with leaves, finely chopped
spinach or chard	2 ounces finely chopped leaves
water	1½ quarts
honey	1 level tbsp
tomato purée	2 tbsp
chives	1 tbsp, finely snipped

Gaylord Hauser was one of the pioneering American naturopaths during the golden era of Hollywood. All the great stars of the 1940s, 1950s, and 1960s flocked to see him. He was an extraordinary man who exuded energy from every pore. He gave me this recipe, which he used in his fasting regimes as an energy booster.

Put the carrots, celery, and spinach or chard into a saucepan with the water. Simmer for 30 minutes. Add the tomato purée and honey and cook for a further 5 minutes. Transfer the soup to a blender or food processor and whiz until smooth. Ladle into soup bowls, sprinkle the snipped chives on top, and serve.

leek and potato soup

extra-virgin olive oil	4 tbsp
leeks	2, large, cleaned, trimmed and roughly chopped
potatoes	1 pound, peeled and cubed
basic chicken stock (see recipe, page 228)	5 cups
flat-leaf parsley	4 tbsp finely chopped leaves, plus extra to garnish
live natural yogurt	2 cups

This traditional soup is a great source of energy thanks to the carbohydrate in the potatoes. Combined with the protection for the heart and circulation given by the leeks, it's an extremely healthful soup as well. For something really different, use sweet potatoes. Their high betacarotene content provides a huge immune boost.

Heat the oil in a large saucepan and sauté the leeks gently for about 10 minutes. Add the potatoes and continue to cook for about 5 minutes. Pour in the stock and simmer until the potatoes are tender, about 15 minutes. Transfer to a blender or food processor and whiz until smooth. Return to the heat, add the parsley, and simmer for 5 minutes. Stir in the yogurt and garnish with the extra parsley.

For a cold version, strain the mixture after it has been whized. Mix in the yogurt, but omit the chopped parsley and garnish with chopped leaves.

corn and haddock chowder

smoked haddock	8 ounces
2 percent milk	3 cups
bay leaves	2
unsalted butter	4 tbsp
onion	1, large, very finely chopped
garlic	1 clove, very finely chopped
potatoes	8 ounces, peeled and finely cubed
frozen or canned corn	1 cup
light cream	1½ cups

At first sight you may wonder what this soup has to offer for radiance, but the fish is a rich source of iodine, lack of which can lead to dry, lifeless hair, coarseness of the skin, and chronic exhaustion. Iodine is also essential for the normal function of the thyroid gland, which controls the body's metabolism, so that's an important bonus.

Poach the haddock in the milk, with the bay leaves, for about 5 minutes. Remove the bay leaves and discard. Remove the fish with a slotted spoon and flake the flesh with a fork. Reserve the poaching liquid. Heat the butter in a saucepan and sauté the onion and garlic gently until soft. Add the potatoes and the reserved poaching liquid and simmer until tender. Add the corn, then stir in the fish and cream and heat through for 5 minutes or until the corn is tender. Serve immediately.

chilled avocado soup

avocados	5, ripe
very veggie stock (see recipe, page 227)	1 quart
lemon	juice of 1
garlic	2 large cloves, finely chopped
red chiles	2, seeded and chopped
cayenne pepper	½ tbsp
green onions	5, roughly chopped
tomatoes	1 cup canned
live natural yogurt	¾ cup
pumpkin seeds	2 tbsp

The ultimate for inner and outer radiance, offering the legendary skin benefits of avocados, which are rich in vitamin E and antioxidants, the circulation-boosting properties of chile and cayenne pepper, the protective bacteria in the yogurt, and lots of zinc from the pumpkin seeds.

Put the avocado flesh into a food processor or large blender with the next 7 ingredients and whiz until smooth. Add the yogurt and whiz again for a few seconds. Spoon into a bowl and let cool in the refrigerator. Dry-fry the pumpkin seeds in a small frying pan. Remove the pan from the heat and let cool. Sprinkle the pumpkin seeds on the soup just before serving.

watercress soup

Watercress is one of the truly great radiance foods. It's hugely anti-oxidant, especially protective against lung cancer, and rich in iron, which makes it a key to inner beauty.

olive oil	1 tbsp
onion	1, finely chopped
garlic	2 cloves, finely chopped
watercress	3 bunches, with stalks
very veggie stock (see recipe, page 227)	1 quart
live natural yogurt	1 cup

Heat the oil in a large saucepan and sauté the onion gently until soft. Add the garlic and continue to cook for 2 minutes. Add the watercress and continue to cook gently until it wilts. Add the stock and simmer for about 10 minutes. Transfer to a blender or food processor and whiz until smooth. Serve hot or cold with a swirl of yogurt in each bowl.

spinach soup with yogurt

canola oil	2 tbsp
onion	1, finely chopped
garlic	2 cloves, finely chopped
fresh or frozen spinach	2 pounds
mint	3 tender sprigs
very veggie stock (see recipe, page 227)	1 quart
live natural yogurt	1 cup
freshly grated nutmeg	4 pinches

Heat the oil in a saucepan and sauté the onion and garlic gently until soft. Add the spinach, mint, and stock and simmer for 10 minutes. Transfer the soup to a blender or food processor and whiz until smooth. Serve with a swirl of yogurt and the nutmeg on top.

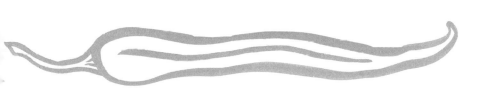

onion soup

The traditional detox soup as well as being sometimes used to relieve bronchitis and other chest infections. What's more, it's a standard French cure for hangovers.

Preheat the broiler and line the broiler pan with foil. Heat the butter in a large saucepan. Add the onions and sauté until just turning golden. Add the flour, mix thoroughly, and cook for 2 minutes. Pour in the stock and thyme and simmer for 10 minutes.

Meanwhile, toast the bread lightly and cut a circle out of each slice. Sprinkle the cheese on top and cook under the preheated grill until the cheese has melted. Serve the soup hot with the cheese-toasted bread floating on top.

unsalted butter	4 tbsp
sweet onions	2, peeled and sliced into rings
all-purpose flour	1 tbsp
very veggie stock (see recipe, page 227)	3¼ cups
thyme	4 large sprigs, leaves finely chopped
whole-wheat bread	4 slices
Gruyère cheese	4 ounces, grated

oat and broccoli soup

This might sound like a cross between breakfast and lunch, but it tastes great. It is extremely cleansing as part of a detox regime and helps protect against heart disease and bowel cancer.

Heat the olive oil in a large saucepan and sauté the green onions gently until just soft. Add the broccoli and continue cooking, stirring continuously, for 2 minutes. Add the oats and stir for 1 minute. Mix together the stock and milk and add to the saucepan. Cover and simmer for 10 minutes. Add the nutmeg. Just before serving, stir in the cream and scatter the chives over the top.

extra-virgin olive oil	2 tbsp
green onions	6, chopped
broccoli	1 pound, cut into florets
uncooked oats	¼ cup
very veggie stock (see recipe, page 227)	2¼ cups
2 percent milk	2¼ cups
nutmeg	½ tsp
light cream	2 tbsp
chives	10, snipped

my salad dressing

extra-virgin olive oil	1½ cups
white wine vinegar	½ cup
Dijon mustard	1 tbsp
green onions	2, very finely chopped
garlic	1 clove, very finely chopped
parsley	1 tsp freshly chopped leaves

Mix all the ingredients together in a bowl. Transfer to a screw-topped jar and shake well. Serve. This will keep for up to 2 weeks, unrefrigerated.

watercress salad

watercress	1 bunch or bag, rinsed (even if the package says it's washed) and all thick stems removed
red onion	1, large, very finely sliced
mint	4 large sprigs, leaves removed and roughly torn
lemon	juice of 1
olive oil	5 tbsp

No one eats enough watercress. It's a good source of iron and vitamin C but, most importantly, it contains chemicals that protect specifically against lung cancer – vital for smokers.

Mix the watercress, onion slices, and mint together in a bowl. Whisk the lemon juice and olive oil together and pour over the salad.

cucumber and strawberry salad

cucumbers	2, large, peeled and very finely sliced
arugula	3 sprigs, leaves finely torn
strawberries	10, large, hulled and cubed
balsamic vinegar	2 tbsp

Put the cucumber into a colander and sprinkle with salt. Leave for about 1 hour so all the water is drawn out. Rinse thoroughly and dry in a clean dish towel. Put the cucumber into a large bowl, add the arugula and strawberries and mix throughly. Sprinkle the balsamic vinegar over the top and serve.

carrot salad

carrots	4, grated
sliced almonds	3 tbsp
raisins	⅓ cup
my salad dressing	½ cup
(see recipe, page 237)	

Mix the first 3 ingredients together in a bowl. Stir in the salad dressing and blend thoroughly. Serve.

tsatsiki

live natural yogurt	1¼ cups
cucumber	1, peeled, seeded and finely grated
garlic	2 cloves, peeled and chopped
mint	5 sprigs, leaves removed, plus 4 sprigs left whole

As well as being good for your digestion, thanks to the mint and bacteria in the yogurt, this also provides calcium for strong bones.

Put all the ingredients except the mint sprigs into a blender. Whiz until smooth. Serve with the mint sprigs on top.

celery salad

celery	8 stalks
capers	4 tsp, rinsed
cottage cheese	½ cup
chives	10, finely snipped

Arrange the celery in 4 bowls. Bruise the capers with the back of a fork, then put them in a bowl, add the cottage cheese, and mix thoroughly. Transfer the mixture to the 4 bowls and serve with the chives sprinkled on top.

fruit crudités with ricotta cheese dip

mixed fresh fruit	about 1 pound, peeled and cored if necessary, but leave apples, peaches, and pears unpeeled
ricotta cheese	1 cup
mint	4 sprigs

Cut the fruit into bite-size pieces and arrange around the edges of 4 large plates. Beat the cheese until smooth and pile in a mound in the middle of each plate. Serve with the mint sprigs garnishing the cheese.

tomato, red onion, and beet salad

beefsteak tomatoes	4, coarsely chopped
red onion	1, coarsely chopped
beets	3, cooked (but not pickled) and diced
beansprouts	7 ounces
my salad dressing (see recipe, page 237)	⅔ cup
coriander	1 small bunch, leaves freshly chopped
mascarpone cheese	½ cup

Mix the first 4 ingredients together, tossing them well in a large bowl. Whisk the dressing, coriander, and mascarpone cheese together in a separate bowl and drizzle it on top. Serve.

grapefruit, peach and mascarpone salad

pink grapefruit	2, peeled and cut into segments
peaches	4, pitted and cut into slices about the size of the grapefruit segments
green onions	4, very finely sliced
mascarpone cheese	1 scant cup

Arrange the grapefruit and peach slices around the sides of a large serving plate. Put the green onions and mascarpone into a blender and whiz until smooth. Drizzle the mascarpone dressing on top of the fruit and serve.

carrot and red cabbage salad

carrots	2, large, grated
red cabbage	½, finely shredded
apples	2, peeled and finely grated
red bell pepper	1, seeded and finely cubed
plum tomatoes	4, quartered
radishes	10, quartered
celery	2 stalks, finely chopped
sunflower seeds	2 tbsp
extra-virgin olive oil	6 tbsp
lemon	juice of ½

This really is health on a plate as it contains enormous amounts of protective carotenoids and cleansing fiber. It also has a gentle diuretic action.

Mix the first 7 ingredients together in a bowl and blend thoroughly. Sprinkle the sunflower seeds on top. Whisk the olive oil and lemon juice together in a separate bowl, drizzle over the salad, and serve.

avocado, tomato, and mushroom salad

avocados	2, peeled, stoned and sliced lengthwise
beefsteak tomatoes	4, sliced widthwise
button mushrooms	4 ounces, wiped and finely sliced
extra-virgin olive oil	about 5 tbsp
limes	juice of 2
black pepper	to serve

Bursting with protective anti-oxidants, especially vitamin E and lycopene, which help prevent some forms of cancer.
Arrange the avocado and tomato slices around the edge of 4 plates. Mix together the mushrooms, oil, and lime juice and pile them in the center of the plates. Serve with a generous grinding of black pepper.

bread and tomato salad

whole-wheat bread	10 medium slices
garlic	4 cloves
extra-virgin olive oil	⅔ cup
plum tomatoes	6, fat, roughly chopped
lemon	juice of 1
mixed fresh herbs	5 tbsp, chopped
black pepper	to taste

Nothing could be a quicker, easier, or more instant source of energy than this typical dish from southern Spain.
Remove the crusts from the bread and cube. Chop the garlic finely. Heat the oil in a large frying pan, add the bread and garlic and toss until all the oil is absorbed and the bread is just beginning to turn golden. Transfer to a salad bowl, add the tomatoes, lemon juice, herbs, and plenty of black pepper. Toss well to serve.

red, white, and green coleslaw

carrots	2, grated
white cabbage	¼
onion	1, small, finely chopped
raisins	4 tbsp
live natural yogurt	1 cup
extra-virgin olive oil	4 tbsp
cider vinegar	1 tbsp
allspice	1 tsp

Mix the vegetables and raisins together in a large serving bowl. Whisk the oil, vinegar, and allspice together and drizzle this dressing over the salad. Mix thoroughly and serve.

spanish salad

tomatoes	1 pound, roughly chopped
bell peppers	2 red, 1 green, seeded and sliced lengthwise
cucumber	1, peeled, seeded and cubed
onion	1, large, sweet, roughly chopped
parsley	10 sprigs, leaves finely chopped
my salad dressing (see recipe, page 237)	½ cup

Just put all the ingredients into a large bowl and toss thoroughly.

tuna and mixed bean salad

tuna	1 x 12-ounce can
mixed beans	2 cups cooked or canned
red onion	1, large, finely chopped
my salad dressing (see recipe, page 237)	½ cup
eggs	2, hard-boiled and quartered
parsley	4 tbsp freshly chopped leaves

This is a perfect lunch if you have a busy afternoon ahead. The beans provide an abundance of instant slow-release energy, and the tuna is an excellent source of easily digested protein to give your brain a boost.

Drain and flake the tuna and drain and rinse the beans. Mix together the fish, beans, and onion. Pour over the salad dressing and mix again. Arrange the eggs on top and scatter the parsley over the salad.

tomato and red onion salad

beefsteak tomatoes	4, finely sliced
onions	2, large, finely sliced
my salad dressing (see recipe, page 237)	½ cup
basil	½ handful roughly torn leaves

Arrange the tomato and onion slices around the sides of the serving plates. Drizzle the dressing on top and sprinkle with the basil leaves. Serve immediately.

papaya and watercress salad

watercress	2 large bunches, thick stems removed
papaya	1, large, peeled, seeds removed and sliced
beefsteak tomatoes	2, large, sliced
lime	juice of 1
cilantro	1 bunch, leaves finely chopped
walnut oil	2 tbsp

An unusual mixture, which tastes as good as it looks. There are energy-stimulating essential oils in the coriander, natural sugars in the tomatoes and papaya, and an abundance of energy-boosting protective chemicals in the watercress.

Put the watercress on a large serving plate. Arrange alternate slices of papaya and tomato on top. Mix together the lime juice, cilantro, and walnut oil and drizzle the dressing on top. Serve immediately.

hummus

chickpeas	1 x 15-ounce can, drained and rinsed
lemon	juice of 1
garlic	2 cloves, peeled and finely grated
mint	3 large sprigs, roughly torn, plus 4 sprigs left whole
extra-virgin olive oil	2 tbsp

Put the first 3 ingredients and the torn mint into a blender or food processor and whiz until blended. Keep the machine running and gradually add the olive oil until the mixture is smooth. Transfer to a serving dish. Garnish with mint sprigs and serve.

guacamole

avocados	2
lemon	juice of 1
live natural yogurt	½ cup
tomatoes	1 cup, canned, drained
garlic	3 cloves, very finely chopped
Tabasco sauce	1 tsp

Mash the avocado flesh and mix thoroughly with the rest of the ingredients. Transfer to a serving dish with the avocado pits – this stops the mixture from going brown. Remove the pits before serving.

avocado, tomato, and mozzarella salad

avocados	2, cubed
cherry tomatoes	8, halved
mozzarella cheese	2 ounces, cubed
chickpeas	1 x 15-ounce can, drained and rinsed
my salad dressing (see recipe, page 237)	½ cup
basil	6 fresh sprigs, leaves roughly torn

Put the first 4 ingredients into a large serving bowl. Pour over the salad dressing and mix well. Scatter the basil leaves on top just before serving.

channel island potato salad

new potatoes	1 pound, 8 ounces
sun-dried tomato paste	3 tbsp
lemon	juice of ½
roasted red peppers	1 x 25-ounce jar, drained
feta cheese	½ cup, cubed
black or green olives	⅓ cup, pitted
basil	2 sprigs, leaves roughly torn

This terrific energy salad has lots of immune-boosting vitamin C, cancer-protective lycopene from the tomato paste, and calcium and protein from the cheese.

Cook the potatoes in a large saucepan of boiling water. Mix together the sun-dried tomato paste and lemon juice. Drain the potatoes and put them, still warm, into a large serving bowl. Add the peppers, cutting them into fine slivers if too large. Pour on the dressing. When the potatoes are cold, add the feta cheese and olives. Scatter the basil leaves on top and serve.

greek salad

tomatoes	8 ounces, quartered
onion	1, finely sliced
green bell pepper	1, seeded and cubed
cucumber	1, peeled, seeded and cubed
black olives	12
feta cheese	½ cup, cubed
extra-virgin olive oil	5 tbsp
oregano	3 tbsp roughly chopped leaves

Every mouthful of this salad just bursts with Mediterranean radiance magic . . . lycopene in the tomatoes, vitamin C in the pepper, calcium in the cheese, and essential oils in the oregano.

Mix the first 6 ingredients together in a large serving bowl. Drizzle over the olive oil and scatter over the oregano leaves.

fava bean, tomato, and herb salad

fava beans	1 pound shelled weight – fresh are best, but frozen will do
plum tomatoes	4, roughly chopped
extra-virgin olive oil	5 tbsp
oregano	2 tbsp roughly chopped leaves

Cook the fava beans in a saucepan of boiling water until tender. Drain, then pinch off the tough thicker skins unless they're very young and leave to cool. Put the tomatoes into a serving bowl, add the broad beans and mix together. Drizzle over the olive oil and sprinkle the chopped oregano over the top.

eggplant caviar with crudités

eggplants	2, large
lemon	juice of 1
extra-virgin olive oil	3 tbsp
garlic	1 clove, very finely chopped
live natural yogurt	1 cup
selection of vegetables – carrots, pepper, celery, cucumber, fennel, cauliflower, and broccoli	raw and cut into fine strips or broken into florets

Eggplant provides high levels of radiant and protective anti-oxidants, and the raw vegetables contain skin-nourishing carotenoids, minerals, and vitamin C.

Preheat the oven to 400°F. Put the eggplants into a large roasting dish and bake in the preheated oven until soft, about 20 minutes. Leave to cool slightly, then cut open and scrape out the flesh. Put the eggplant flesh into a bowl and add the lemon juice. Gradually beat in the oil and mix in the garlic and yogurt. Serve as a dip with the raw vegetables.

salad vegeçoise

Radiance on a plate, thanks to the skin-nourishing betacarotene in the peppers, the B vitamins in the eggs, and all the natural oils in the olives.

Iceberg lettuce	1, large, roughly shredded
cucumber	½, peeled, seeded and sliced
red bell pepper	1, seeded and cubed
tomatoes	6, quartered and seeded
eggs	4, hard-boiled and quartered
black olives	12, pitted
my salad dressing (see recipe, page 237)	½ cup

Put the lettuce into a large, wide bowl. Arrange the other salad vegetables on top. Place the eggs and olives around the side of the bowl. Pour the dressing over the salad and serve.

crudités with garlic mayonnaise

egg yolks	3
garlic	3 large cloves, pressed or minced
salt	a pinch
extra-virgin olive oil	1½ cups
lemon	juice of 1 small
selection of vegetables – carrots, pepper, celery, cucumber, fennel, cauliflower and broccoli	raw and cut Into fine strips or broken into florets

Put the eggs yolks and garlic into a blender with a pinch of salt. Whiz until the yolks are frothy. With the machine still running, add the oil in a fine stream and the lemon juice a little at a time. Transfer to a serving bowl. Serve as a dip with the raw vegetables.

carrot and melon salad

carrots	3
galia melons	2
sesame seeds	2 tbsp
my salad dressing (see recipe, page 237)	½ cup

Peel and coarsely grate the carrots and peel, seed, and cube the melons. Mix together the carrots and melon. Dry fry the sesame seeds in a small frying pan until just changing color. Remove from the heat and let cool slightly. Pour over the carrots and melon. Drizzle over the dressing and serve.

desserts

spiced baked apples

ground almonds	2 tbsp
raisins	1 tbsp
orange juice	1 tbsp
cooking apples	4, washed, cored and with the bottom ½ inch of the core replaced
cloves	4
unsalted butter	4 tbsp
brown sugar	1 tbsp
freshly ground nutmeg	4 pinches

The simple addition of ground almonds and raisins adds valuable energy-giving calories and a host of other essential and radiance-boosting nutrients to this simple dessert.

Preheat the oven to 375°F. Mix together the almonds, raisins, and orange juice. Spoon into the cored cavities of the apples. Top each one with a clove. Use half the butter to grease a large ovenproof dish and the other half to smear over the apple skins. Place the apples in the dish, sprinkle over the sugar and nutmeg, and bake in the preheated oven for 25 minutes.

dried fruit compôte

prunes	½ cup, pitted
dried apricots	½ cup
dried figs	⅔ cup
raisins	¼ cup
rosehip teabags	2
honey	2 tbsp
cloves	4
live natural yogurt	1½ cups
lemon	grated zest of 1
ground cinnamon	1 tsp
sliced almonds	2 tbsp

Wash the fruit under cold running water and put into a large bowl with the teabags, honey, and cloves. Cover completely with freshly boiled water, stir, and let cool. Remove the teabags and strain the fruit into 2 bowls. Mix the yogurt, lemon zest, and cinnamon in a separate bowl. Serve the fruit with the yogurt sauce on top and sprinkled with the almonds.

honeyed plums

red plums	1 pound, washed but left whole
honey	2 tbsp
red wine	4 tbsp
cardamom pods	6
brandy	1 tbsp
mascarpone cheese	1 cup

Put the plums, honey, wine, and cardamom pods into a large saucepan, cover and simmer until the plums begin to break up, about 8–10 minutes. Add the brandy and heat through for 1 minute. Transfer to serving bowls and serve with the mascarpone cheese.

banana and mango crumble

mango	1, large, cubed
bananas	4, peeled and thickly sliced
lemon	juice and grated rind of 1
soft brown sugar	2 tbsp
whole-wheat breadcrumbs	4 ounces
unsalted butter	8 tbsp
muesli	⅔ cup, organic

Yes, this crumble is made with butter, but there really isn't an alternative, so don't even try to think of one. It provides lots of energy, plus plenty of potassium from the bananas and loads of betacarotene from the mango. And it's delicious.

Preheat the oven to 375°F. Mix together the mango, bananas, lemon juice and rind, and half the sugar. Pour into a lightly greased pie plate. Mix together the breadcrumbs and 6 tablespoons of the butter. Add the rest of the sugar and the muesli. Mix thoroughly and pour evenly over the top of the fruit. Dot with the rest of the butter and cook in the preheated oven for 20 minutes.

orange and mango fool

mangoes	2, ripe, peeled and cubed
orange	juice and grated rind of 1 small
live natural yogurt	1 cup

Put all the ingredients into a blender or food processor and whiz until smooth. Spoon into serving bowls, chill, then serve.

mango and kiwi sorbet

brown pourable sugar	1 cup
rosewater	1 cup
kiwi fruit	2, peeled and cubed
mango	1, ripe, peeled and cubed
mint	8 leaves, roughly torn
egg white	1

Boil the sugar and rosewater for 1 minute until the sugar is dissolved. Remove from the heat and let cool. Put the fruit and mint into a blender or food processor and whiz until smooth. Add the rosewater syrup and egg white and whiz again. Pour into a shallow, freezer-proof container and put in the freezer until almost solid. Take out, break up with a fork, and return to the freezer until solid again. Leave at moderate room temperature for 20 minutes before serving.

spiced apricots

dried apricots	1 cup
cloves	4
allspice	½ tsp
apple juice	1½ cups
honey	1 tbsp
cinnamon	1 small stick
freshly grated nutmeg	½ tsp
orange	grated peel of 1

Put all the ingredients into a large saucepan. Bring to the boil, turn down the heat, and simmer until the apricots are tender, about 20 minutes. Remove the cinnamon stick before serving.

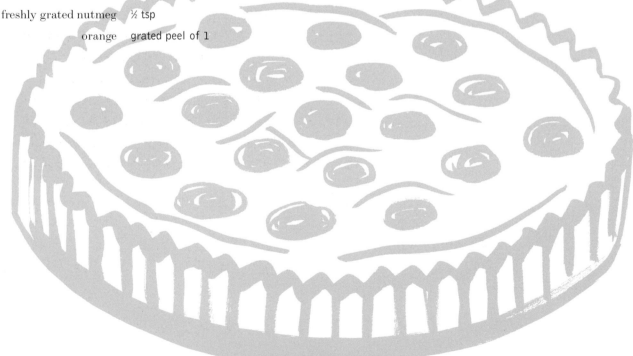

apricot and almond crumble

unsalted butter	4 tbsp, cut into small cubes
apricots	6, pitted and halved
turbinado sugar	2 tbsp
uncooked oats	1 cup
ground almonds	4 tbsp
honey	1 tbsp
sliced almonds	3 tbsp

Don't feel guilty about enjoying this delicious pudding. After all, feeling good is a major factor in looking good, and enjoyment of any sort helps you feel good. On top of that, apricots are a major source of vitamin A, almonds provide vitamin E and essential minerals, and oats are rich in the B vitamins. So this is a really sweet treat.

Preheat the oven to 400°F. Use about half the butter to grease a pie dish. Add the apricots, sugar, and 2 tbsp of water. Mix the oats and ground almonds together in a bowl and sprinkle over the top. Drizzle with the honey. Scatter over the almonds and dot with the rest of the butter. Bake in the preheated oven for 20 minutes.

fresh cherry tarts

puff pastry	1 sheet
fresh cherries	1 pound, pitted
eggs	2
live natural yogurt	1 cup
superfine sugar	2 tbsp
cherry brandy	2 tbsp

As well as skin-nourishing protective anti-oxidants and masses of vitamin C, cherries contain substantial quantities of bio-flavonoids, which slow down the aging process of the skin.

Preheat the oven to 425°F. Grease 4 individual springform tart pans, roll out the pastry, divide into 4 and use to line the tart pans. Put the cherries on top of the pastry. Beat the eggs together in a bowl. Put the yogurt, half the sugar, and the cherry brandy into a bowl and beat in the eggs. Pour the mixture over the cherries, scatter the remaining sugar on top, and bake in the preheated oven for 25 minutes, or until the filling has risen and turned a golden color.

eggs	4
brown pourable sugar	4 tsp
oranges	juice and grated rind of 2
unsalted butter	2 tbsp
confectioners' sugar	1 tbsp

orange soufflé omelette

Separate the egg yolks from the whites. Beat the yolks, then add the sugar, orange juice and rind and mix together. Put the egg whites into a spotlessly clean bowl and whisk into peaks. Fold the egg whites into the yolk mixture. Melt the butter in a nonstick frying pan, pour in a quarter of the mixture and cook the omelette. When it begins to bubble, put the pan under a preheated hot broiler to puff up and turn brown. Dust with confectioners' sugar to serve. Repeat to make the remaining omelettes.

summer fruits	2 pounds – use thawed frozen fruit if it's the middle of winter
heavy cream	1 cup
live natural yogurt	1 cup
brown pourable sugar	4 tbsp

fresh fruit brûlée

All the summer fruits just ooze super nutrients and they are right up there at the top of the inner and outer radiance list. Yes, this is made with heavy cream – but you aren't going to eat it every day.

Preheat the broiler. Put the fruit into a large soufflé dish. Beat the cream, then mix in the yogurt. Spread the mixture over the fruit and sprinkle the sugar on top. Put the dish under the preheated grill for 4 minutes until the top is golden. Serve immediately.

pink grapefruit sorbet

superfine sugar	1 cup
rosewater	1 cup
pink grapefruit juice	1¼ cups
lemon	juice of 1
pink grapefuit	1, peeled and segmented

Boil the sugar and rosewater for 5 minutes, remove the pan from the heat, and let cool. Mix with the grapefruit and lemon juices and transfer to a freezing container. Put in the freezer until almost firm. Remove from the freezer, break up with a fork, and freeze again. Remove from the freezer 20 minutes before serving and put in the refrigerator. Serve garnished with the grapefruit segments.

stewed pears with mascarpone and cloves

firm pears	1 pound, peeled, cored and sliced
sugar	2 tbsp
cloves	4
mascarpone cheese	1 generous cup

Put the pears, sugar, and cloves in a large saucepan with 4 tbsp of water and cook gently. When they are cooked, remove the cloves and discard. Stir in the mascarpone cheese and leave to cool before serving.

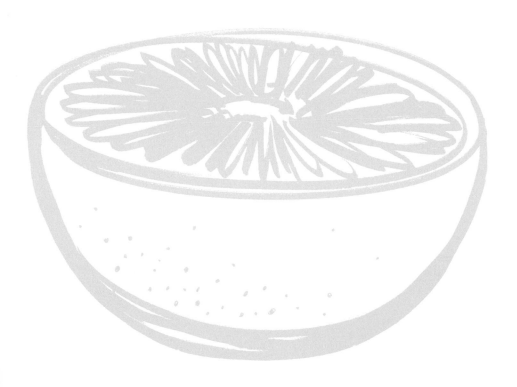

index

picture credits

1 Gettyimages/V.C.L/Paul Viant; 2-3 Digital Vision; 6-7 Digital Vision; 12-13 Gettyimages/Paul Stanier; 15 Gettyimages/V.C.L/Bronwyn Ridd; 22 Digital Vision; 24-25 Digital Vision; 27 Digital Vision; 30-31 Gettyimages/Garry Hunter; 39 Diana Miller; 41 Digital Vision; 46-47 Digital Vision; 49 Digital Vision; 52 Digital Vision; 55 Gettyimages/Sarto-Lund; 58 Gettyimages/Peter Holst; 60-61 Gettyimages/Erlanson Productions; 62-63 Digital Vision; 68-69 Digital Vision; 71 Gettyimages/Bill Losh; 81 Digital Vision; 82 Digital Vision; 87 Digital Vision; 96 Zefa Visual Media UK Ltd/E. Holub; 101 Gettyimages/Dennis O'Clair; 111 Gettyimages/Deborah Jaffe; 112-113 Digital Vision; 115 Gettyimages/Michael Goldman; 117 Digital Vision; 118 Digital Vision; 120-121 Gettyimages/Laurence Monneret; 126-127 Gettyimages/Mark Wright; 129 Gettyimages/Dennie Cody; 132 Digital Vision; 136-137 Gettyimages/John Burwell; 141 Gettyimages/Szczepaniak; 150 Gettyimages/Adrian Neal; 153 Gettyimages/Alan Powdrill; 155 Gettyimages/Michelangelo Gratton; 156 Gettyimages/Candice Farmer; 168-169 Gettyimages/Scott Morgan; 170-171 Gettyimages/David Rosenberg; 174-175 Digital Visionz

Answers to anagrams	Answers to mental maths
1 Parliament	1 112
2 Clint Eastwood	2 11
3 Mental energy	3 48
4 Super energy detox	4 6
5 Exodus	5 143
6 Beefburger	6 1000
7 Brainstorming	7 4,777,800

Editorial Director: Jane O'Shea
Consultant Art Director: Françoise Dietrich
Art Editor: Rachel Gibson
Project Editor: Hilary Mandleberg
Production: Nancy Roberts
Illustrations: Janet Simon

First published in 2003 by
Quadrille Publishing Limited
Alhambra House
27–31 Charing Cross Road
London WC2H 0LS

This edition published in the US and Canada
by Whitecap Books Ltd. For more information,
please contact Whitecap Books,
351 Lynn Avenue, North Vancouver,
British Columbia, Canada V7J 2C4

British Library Cataloguing-in-Publication Data
A catalogue record for this book is available from the
British Library.

ISBN 1-55285-545-7
Printed in Spain